VigorRobic®

MW00571643

To my parents

Remarks:
Always consult a physician before you start a new physical program. If you have any physical defects and take medication, this is absolutely necessary. Neither author nor publishing house is liable for consequential damages.

VigorRobic® a registered trademark.

Expression of thanks:
I thank Reebok Germany GmbH for providing the clothing, shoes, small tools and accessories.

I also thank Monika Liening, owner of Ladyfitness Untereschach and the two owners of the fitness-center Refrath, "the Fitmaker" for letting me use their studios.

Frank Sommer

*Vigor**Robic**®*

Increased Potency through Specific Fitness Training

Meyer & Meyer Sport

Original title: VigorRobic®
Aachen: Meyer und Meyer Verlag, 2000
Translated by Anja Haudricourt

British Library Cataloguing in Publication Data
A catalogue for this book is available from the British Library

Sommer, Frank:
VigorRobic®/Frank Sommer
– Oxford: Meyer und Meyer, (UK) Ltd., 2002
ISBN 1-84126-078-9

© 2002 by Meyer & Meyer Sport (UK) Ltd.
Aachen, Adelaide, Auckland, Budapest, Graz, Johannesburg,
Miami, Olten (CH), Oxford, Singapore, Toronto
Member of the World
Sports Publishers' Association
www.w-s-p-a.org

Printed and bound by Vimperk AG
ISBN 1-84126-078-9
E-Mail: verlag@meyer-meyer-sports.com
www.meyer-meyer-sports.com

Contents

Introduction

Keeping your potency and increasing it has always been a topic of interest. And it will always be like this, too. Generations of people before our time have faced up to this subject. Our children, grandchildren and great-grandchildren will also do this. The constantly erected Phallus of Priapos, one of the gods of fertility from antiquity, back then already was a symbol of strength, power, potency and fertility. The subject of the male sexuality has always been a part of the history of human beings, with a few up and downs in its topicality up to now in our highly industrial time. Let us not forget that this subject is treated very differently in different cultures, states and societies. The question of the sexual potency of the man reached a new high at the beginning of 1998 when Viagra®, the "blue wonderpill" was placed for sale on the American market. The press, radio and TV, and last but not least the men, pushed this perpetual subject back to position no. 1.

Where are we at the moment? – In our western culture and bourgeois society especially activity, aggressiveness, self-control and strength are the adjectives used for a man, all these are considered when estimating his sexual drive. This is the reason why the self-esteem and the self-confidence of a man who is not always "ready" – not to talk about him being impotent – is very crushed. To be impotent for the person concerned does not only mean that he will encounter problems with regard to his relationships but also often means being a failure in the professional, social and family role. A vicious cycle between failing and reduction of self-esteem can develop from this.

A man does not speak about having problems with his sexual potency, nobody wants to expose oneself, but potency and the result of potency increasing methods are excessively talked about. Many myths are haunting within our heads and in the press. Most so called potency increasing measures lack any kind of well-grounded information. Some medications do have an effect at the place where the success is supposed to come, but they also have strong physical side-effects and, due to their price, lead to financial losses.

It is known that virility decreases when getting older. The circulation, the elasticity of the tissue and the ability to keep the blood in the penis during an erection decreases. In an extensive study in the US it was determined that 52% of all American men between the age of 40 and 70 are fighting unwanted problems of potency.

Juveniles can also suffer from impaired potency, for example caused by a period of sexual inactivity or through a general weak definition of the structures that cause the erection.

One often knows subconsciously that certain activities or movements cause a certain reaction in the body. But there is a lack of a medical and natural scientific background knowledge to explain this phenomenon.

As a urologist as well as a sports physician, I have intensively studied the effects of sports on potency. The laymen's press as well as medical journals reported a connection between impotence and cycling sports. In my first studies I did some research on this connection. The circulation of the penis of bicycle riders was checked during the whole sport activity. While sitting on the racing saddle, the circulation was strongly decreased! Now the question was raised how to avoid this effect. Studies were performed using different postures.

During cycling tours of medium strain in a standing position as well as when cycling on a recumbent bicycle, the circulation of blood in the penis was not decreased. But who is able to constantly cycle in a standing position? Or what are you supposed to do if no recumbent bicycle is available? From this point of view, the question comes up whether there are exercises to promote the circulation of the penis – as a kind of compensation training.

They do exist! I have found out that a certain way of muscle training and a special method to exercise endurance increases the blood circulation in the penis. But why should only bicycle riders perform these exercises and training programs that increase the blood circulation?

This positive effect resulting from training should be made available to all men. Examinations also have shown that a good oxygen supply of the male genitalia is important to preserve the elasticity of the penis and its structures. Therefore I am working very extensively on coming up with exercise and training programs which increase the oxygen-support as well as the circulation of the penis. The next question I then have asked myself was: What is important in order to get a good erection? The answer: Exercising the steadiness! Now only exercises reducing the circulation back out of the erected penis were still needed.

I found out all three factors that are necessary for a good erection and thus a satisfying sexual life can be exercised. Considering this scientifically acquired knowledge, I developed the training program **VigorRobic®**. This new form of training, **VigorRobic®**, offers possibilities of increasing the blood and oxygen supply and improving the stability of the penis. By this potency will be maintained and increased.

Why should men neglect their potency if they are given the possibility to train it now?

■■ **VigorRobic®** keeps the virility up and even increases it!
■ A pleasant "side-effect" of this training-method:
   The ejaculation can willingly be delayed!
■ Since the mind has a substantial influence on the ability to have a good sex-life, there is another advantage:
   Targeted **VigorRobic®** training increases self-confidence!

11

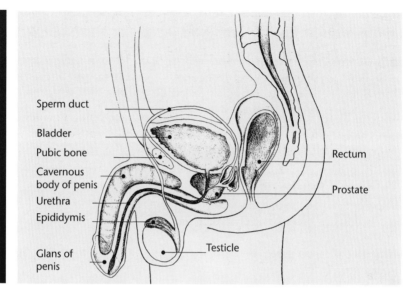

Figure 1: The structure of the male genitalia

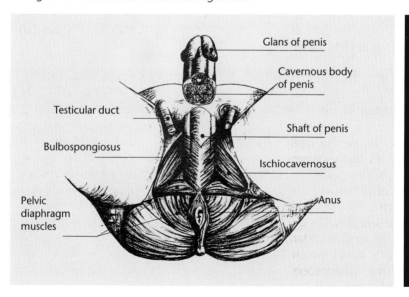

Figure 2: Pelvic diaphragm

PART I – BASICS

1 Anatomy of the Male Genital Organs

To get a better understanding of the ability to exercise the potency and the erection-process, a basic knowledge of the organic structure (anatomy) of the male genital organs is necessary.

The male anatomy *(figure 2)* is separated in external – visible – and internal – not visible – genital organs.

1.1 External Genital Organs

Penis (membrum) and testicular bag (scrotum) build the external male genital organs.

The whole manifold structure of the penis is determined by the ability to get an erection, to impregnate a woman (for the purpose of reproduction) and to urinate (pass water). Contrary to some species of animals, it consists only of different tissues, meaning it does not have osseous or cartilaginous structures.

This tissue is made from two parallel placed cavernous bodies that are only partly separated by a thin elastic wall and therefore enable the exchange of blood in both cavernous bodies. They start at the pelvic diaphragm and skeleton where they are embodied as the so called penis roots above the freely moveable shaft of the penis up to the glans. Muscles (ischiocavernosus and bulbospongiosus, *figure 2*) connect the root of the penis (base) to the pubic bone. Below these pairs of cavernous bodies and in the middle is the individual spongy body of the urethra, which at its outer end builds the glans. The urethra is used for passage of urine and to guide sperm to the outside during the ejaculation. The glans is very sensitive. Many nerves end in it – especially the nerve (nervus dorsalis penis) which is placed above the cavernous bodies –, which transmit information about the process of the erection and the ejaculation over the spinal cord to the brain.

The pairs of cavernous bodies that from the inside look like puffy honeycombed plexus, are filled with blood when the circulation increases and in this way cause the erection. The small, hollow space-like arranged honeycombs are surrounded by nets from connective tissue and smooth muscle cells. When not erected, the screwdriver-like vessels (arterioles), which end in the honeycombed hollow spaces are very tight.

The screwdriver-like structure of the small vessels is important because these vessels are being stretched when the penis is erected, causing an extension (elongation) of the penis. In order for the penis not to be able to extend endlessly, the cavernous bodies are surrounded by a tight, hardly extensible cover (tunica albuginea) from connective tissue which causes the tightening (fixation) during the erection.

In the cavernous bodies end two vessels, in pairs (penis arteries), which are responsible for the blood supply of the male genitalia. These four penis arteries each originate in the pelvic vessels that are also arranged as pairs (Pudendae internae). In addition to that there are nerves (nervi cavernosi penis) in the cavernous bodies, which give electrical commands to the surrounding tissue.

The draining of blood from the hollow space-like arranged honeycombs is regulated by cathartic blood vessels (penis veins) and takes place in a venous network. The complete venous network widens in a non-erected state and the blood can flow through it without any problems. When in a state of erection however, the hollow places are filled with blood and the cathartic blood flow decreases. Above the cavernous bodies are vessels that are ensuring the blood supply and the drainage to the glans and the skin of the penis *(figure 3)*.

The skin of the penis, which is built from two parts (foreskin) close to the glans, covers all of the penis structures, for example the cavernous bodies, the vessels, the nerves and the connective tissue wrap. It is located loosely around the penis and is normally very mobile. The structure which covers the glans is called foreskin and can normally be pulled back easily from the glans; usually this automatically happens during an erection. The inner leaf of the foreskin is in direct contact with the glans and is tightly attached to it through a little bond (small ligament). In it are some glands that discharge a secretion to moisten the attached structures.

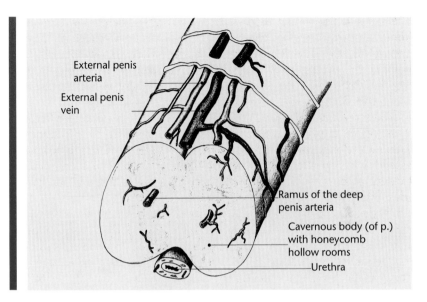

Figure 3: Cross-sectional view of the penis (vascular supply)

Due to a lack of hygiene, white segments can build up which can result in cheese-like concentrated structures.

The testicular scrotum, which contains both testicles, is a kind of bag from the abdominal skin. This structure is full of muscle cells. Stimulations like coldness or a touch can cause the testicular bag to strongly tighten. When doing so, the testicles are pushed upwards towards the abdomen.

There are many nerve endings in the skin of the scrotum meaning it reacts very sensitively to stimulations from the outside.

1.2   Internal Genital Organs

The testicle, the epididymis, the sperm duct, the seminal vesicles and the prostate gland (prostata) are the inner genital organs.

The testicles (genital glands) have the form of a plum and are laid out in pairs. They are of a tight elasticity and are around 4-5 cm long. Often the right testicle is a little larger than the left one and goes a little deeper in the scrotum. The organ is connected with a strong membrane. Among other things, this can cause the intrinsic pressure that is necessary for the production of sperm. The testicles are surrounded by numerous albugineas (layers around the testicle) that have developed from the abdominal membrane. These are very sensitive, which explains the strong pain resulting from pressure on the testicles.

In special cells of the testicle the male genital hormone, testosterone, is produced and when becoming sexually mature, sperm is formed. Since different types of cells are responsible for the hormonogenesis and the spermiogenesis, disturbances can have different effects on both systems. If the quality of the semen is not perfect, this does not necessary have an influence on the male hormones and outward male appearance or even potency.

Through a connection the sperm gets into the testicle and the epididymis and from there further into the sperm duct. Only during the move from the testicle to the sperm duct does the semen get into a stadium of fertility. This on average takes two to three months. For the maturation process it is also important that the testicles lie in the scrotum and not in the abdominal cavity because in order for the semen to mature correctly there has to be a difference in temperature (cooler) to the abdominal cavity. Adults with an inguinal testis, meaning the genital gland cannot be felt in the scrotum, which has not (or too late) been treated in childhood, can suffer from infertility.

The epididymis is in the back of the testicle like a hood. If you feel the testicle on its backside, you can feel it as a tail-like rough structure. The epididymis is made from multiple, crossing corridors. By movement the sperms mature. If the epididymis is strongly infected, the corridors can stick close or even get destroyed. Then the sperms from the infected side of the epididymis cannot get into the sperm duct anymore. This explains why a strong infection of both sides can cause fertility problems. The sperm duct starts at the lower end of the epididymis and further on connects with the urethra. The sperm duct can be easily felt as a rough, solid structure in the testicle. Its wall is made from layers of muscles and connective tissue. During a male sterilisation, the sperm duct is cut and tied up so the sperm cannot be transported any further. The sperm duct that originates from the tail of epididymis goes up into the groin together with tissues and nerves. Inside the pelvis the sperm duct and most vessels

16

and nerves are separated again. The uretal (connection of the kidney with the bladder) is crossed and it goes behind the bladder through the prostate and meets the back urethra at the seminal crest. During the ejection the sperms, that have been mixed with liquid of the seminal vesicle and fluid from the prostate go to the back urethra. From there they are transported outside by the contraction of the urethra.

After a sterilisation the looks and the amount of semen ejaculated hardly ever change because the main part comes from fluid and liquid from the seminal vesicle and the prostate. These fluids and liquids are very important for the movement of the sperm within the female inner genitalia. The sperm get their energy to move and penetrate the egg cells from it.

The seminal vesicles are on the ground of the bladder and are pointed steeply upward. In it sugar (fructose) is produced which is needed for the movement of the sperm. The contents of the seminal vesicles flow – just like the sperm - into the back part of the urethra and are 60-80 % of the ejaculation.

The prostate (prostate gland) is an organ about the size of a chestnut that lies on the ground (base) of the bladder. It consists of three lobars (two side lobars, one middle lobar) and surrounds the urethra after leaving the bladder. The secretory ducts of two grey-yellow structures (Cowper's glands) about the size of peas go parallel to the urethra for a couple of centimetres and then blend in it. Right before the ejaculation its fluid is pressed out through the surrounding muscles and prepares the urethra for the upcoming ejaculation by making it more smooth.

We differentiate numerous zones in the prostate that surround the urethra like peels of an onion. The inner part often begins to grow benignly starting from the age of 40 that can lead to a confinement of the urethra. This again when getting older can lead to problems when urinating. If there are problems to urinate with residual urine formation or if the urine stream is really weak – from drops to not being able to go at all – the inner prostate growth should be surgically removed provided a medical therapy was not successful. Depending on the size of this organ, the removal can be performed through the urethra or by a lower abdominal cut.

A malignant growth, in this case often at the outer part of the gland, is called prostate cancer (carcinoma). Because it is located in the outer part, a hardening can be felt. Health insurances recommend regular preventive examinations starting from 40 years up because at the initial stage when the cancer has no metastases and the malignant growth is only on the prostate it can be removed well by surgery. Prostate cancer is the second most common cancerous growth for male.

2 How Does Erection and Ejaculation Work?

The erection (stiffening of the penis) depends upon a variety of external (exogenous) as well as internal (endogenous) factors. Often it is caused by erotic stimulant, for example optical (erotic movies, pictures, the view of a naked woman or fantasies) or tactile stimulant (meaning information which is transmitted when touching the genitals or the so-called erogenous zones). Here significant individual differences exist. Some men only get a full erection by a manual (using the hand) stimulation of the partner; for others thinking about female forms is sufficient.

The individual differences depend on the individual development, for example the influence when growing up or the first sexual experiences of the individual man. Often the penis hardens without erotic stimulation. A healthy man has erection every $1–1^1/2$ hours while he is sleeping in the phase when his eyes are moving back and forth very fast (rapid eye movement phase). Also when getting up most men have a so-called morning erection.

Internal factors like nerve related ones (neurological), hormonal, arterial (blood supply), venous (blood outflow), but partly also mental (psychic) factors are responsible for a normal erection process.

A normal erection process can be regarded as the response to
■ an increased blood supply (arterial increase of the perfusion) with
■ a decreased blood outflow (venous outflow),

caused by nerve impulses, based on different stimuli including psychic factors like audio-visual observations/perceptions and lust (libido).

I will show you during the course of the book how you can train increasing the blood-supply, a result of which is an increase of the oxygen-supply of the local penile tissue, and how you can lower the blood outflow with the help of **VigorRobic®**.

19

2.1 Phases of Erection

The erection process is separated into different phases:

2.1.1 Limp Phase

In this phase the blood supply as well as the blood outflow is low. The supporting blood vessels are tightened, the smooth muscles are tense (contracted) and therefore it is not possible for the blood to fill the hollow rooms *(figure 4)*. The blood in the penis has little oxygen and equals the used (venous) blood that flows to the heart.

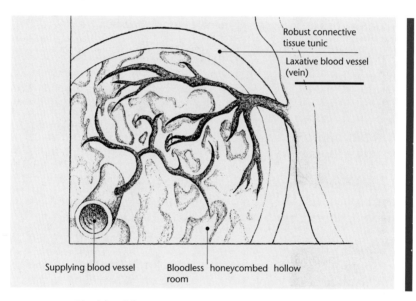

Robust connective tissue tunic

Laxative blood vessel (vein)

Supplying blood vessel

Bloodless honeycombed hollow room

Figure 4: The blood flow in the penis during the "limp phase"

2.1.2 Latent (Filling) Phase

For most men, the visually received erotic stimuli are sent to the brain via the spinal cord to the nerves in the penis. Different substances (neurotransmitters) are set free at the nerve ends. This results in a high blood supply in the penis. The speed of the blood flow increases by 200%, the diameter of the supporting vessels significantly increases. The honeycombed hollow-room structures are filled with blood and the penis starts to enlarge.

2.1.3 Phase of Tumescence (Enlargement of the Penis)

At the same time as the blood supply increases, the blood outflow reduces *(figure 5)*. The volume of the penis and its length significantly increases. The oxygen supply in the penis is at its maximum. The internal penis pressure increases. The blood supply decreases with the increase of the pressure.

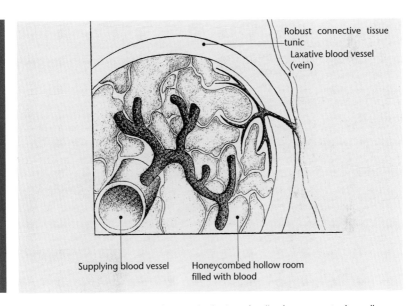

Figure 5: The blood flow in the penis during the "enlargement phase"

2.1.4 Phase of the Full Erection

There is a further reduction of the blood-outflow.
  The resistance of the draining pipes increases about a 100 times more than normal. This is caused by the compression of the draining vessels due to maximum contraction of the pelvic bottom muscles.

2.1.5 Phase of the Hard Erection (Maximum Penis Stiffening)

The pressure is further increased in the cavernous body of the penis resulting in the penis becoming totally stiff and sticking up straight from the body. The blood supply now is minimised because the heart can hardly get over the pressure in the penis to pump more blood into it. The pelvic bottom muscles, especially the ischiocavernosus muscles are flexed to the max and prevent the draining of the blood. Within a short time the penis now is erected to its maximum. It then can be penetrated into the vagina without a problem and sexual intercourse (coitus) can take place.

A further overstimulation of the penis, caused especially by friction of the penis in the vagina, further impulses (signals) are sent via the penis nerves to the spinal marrow. The erection and ejaculation centre is located in the spinal marrow. This is where, later on, the so-called ejaculation reflex is started.

2.1.6 Phase of Detumescence (Relaxation)

Once the erotic stimuli get less or after the ejaculation, the nerve impulses are reduced. The smooth muscles of the cavernous body tighten. Most of the blood is pushed out of the penis. The blood supply and outflow becomes normal again and the penis becomes slack. Length and size of the penis return to normal. Only after a certain time of regeneration after the ejaculation a new erection can follow. The individual regeneration time varies greatly and clearly depends upon the age. It can last between 10 minutes and a couple of days.

2.2 The Ejaculation Process

Emission and ejaculation are the climax of the male sex life. Right before the ejaculation the emission takes place, here the sperm together with the fluid and the secretions from the seminal vesicle and prostate at the seminal crest are emptied into the back urethra. Now the ejaculation reflex follows and cannot be interrupted anymore, squirting the sperm out.

For the man, the ejaculation is the phase of orgasm which usually only lasts a few seconds. Right before the ejaculation, the testicles are moved up towards the perineal region. During the ejaculation the muscles of the bulbospongiosus (BS), ischiocavernousus (IC), the sphincter muscle of the urethra, the bottom of the pelvis as well as the muscles of the ductus deferens, seminal vesicle and prostate tighten. Rhythmic co-ordinated spasms of the urethra pump out the semen by jerks. Right before the ejaculation the bladder muscle tightens at the portal of the bladder, so the sperm does not go back (retrograde) into the bladder.

3 What are the Reasons for Potency Problems

Impaired potency is the most common male sexual malfunction. We make a distinction between:
- the inability to have sex because the penis does not function
- the lack of sexual desire (libido)
- problems with the ejaculation or the orgasm; premature ejaculation (ejaculatio retardata) and the orgasm without an ejaculation (retrograde ejaculation) and
- problems with fertility.

The above mentioned problems can either appear individually or in a combination.

In the 1970s as psycho-therapeutic medicine started to become more established, it was said that 90% of all male sexual malfunctions were due to psychological problems. Because at this time neither the structure of the penis nor its function was understood, impotency was a white spot on the map. Courageous scientists started to discover at least parts of this spot. New examination techniques and therapeutic measures appeared, were given an ovation and were partly thrown away again. At the beginning of the 1990s it was thought that men had problems getting an erection due to organic causes.

During the course of their life, about 50% of all men experience a temporary episode of inability to have sex. 15-25% of all men who consult a physician talk about sexual problems. Chronic erection problems are significantly increasing when getting older. At the age of 60 one fourth already suffer from permanent impotence.

It is well known and almost trite to mention that a lot of different factors play a role with impotence. These symptoms can have totally different causes for the individual patient. In principle, primary malfunctions with potency can be differentiated from secondary. Primary malfunctions become obvious when first becoming sexually active. With secondary malfunctions there is a period of an undisturbed sex life and impotency does not become a factor until later on in life.

3.1 What Is Impotence?

Impotence is a term bearing strong negative associations. It is looked at as a handicap of the man. Medically one speaks about an erectile dysfunction or impaired erection ability, a disorder, not a handicap. Impotency is defined as the inability to get a sufficient stiffness of the penis to have sex. This does not mean the short-termed "failure" of a man but the erectile dysfunction of a longer duration. Some men and couples can handle this situation really well. Only when the person concerned or the relationship of the two suffers from this condition one can talk about an impotence that has to be medically examined.

Problems with sexuality can harm an intact relationship and can even be the reason for split-ups. This especially is the case in new relationships in which sex often plays a more important role than it does in longer lasting relationships. Sexuality does not always take first part in relationships but often it plays an important part in a well-balanced, harmonic relationship. A constant lack of it can cause tension between the partners and be a strong burden on the relationship.

As mentioned before, impotence can have multiple reasons. Below the different possible causes are dealt with individually.

3.2 Mental (Psychogenic) Reasons

In the 1970s one assumed that almost all erection problems were due to mental problems. In the meantime one can determine very clearly between mental and organic problems as well as a mix of both. 15-60% of all men suffer from psychogenic problems. In many cases it becomes a mixture of both. When suffering from impotence due to physical reasons, usually the mental factors start to play a significant role, as well after "failing" a couple of times.

The detailed and skillful check of the medical history (anamnesis) of a patient suffering from erection dysfunction can often point towards the right direction whether there is an organic defect or a psychogenic dysfunction. If the patient talks about erections in the morning, this points towards a psychogenic reason. Furthermore, reports about good stiffening of the penis when watching erotic movies, pornographic photos or masturbating are pointing towards a mental problem for it seems that the penis is functioning well. This means that all organic functions needed for an erection are intact. Impotence is a complex clinical picture and sometimes it is possible only after detailed, intensive examinations to determine whether it is a psychogenic or physical dysfunction.

The causes of psychogenic impotence can include many factors, meaning it can be very different. In addition to psychogenic problems of the man concerned, partner-related factors, especially mechanism of fear of failure and defence because of fear as well as mechanisms of excessive control and self-observation play a decisive role.

In the following we will consider the possible causes of the mental erection dysfunction briefly.

3.2.1 The Problem with the Length of the Penis

Is the problem with the length of the penis not always a psychological problem? No, there are also organic cases. The medically defined micro penis or the strong curvature of the erected penis that can lead to a shortening of it, are organic problems. But we do not want to talk about this subject further.

Many men think that their penis is not long enough. Unfortunately this opinion is as widely spread as it is unfounded. Young people who are not successful during their first sexual experiences (for example if their partner does not get an orgasm) see the reason for this in their apparently too small penis.

Also many older patients complained that their sexual organs have shrunk in the past years. When putting on a lot of weight this can have the effect of a so-called abdominal apron. This does not lead to a shortening of the length of the erectile organ but when the penis is erected it seems to be smaller optically because the fat tissue covers part of it. Many men who consult a physician because of their too small penis know the length of it up to the millimetre. Unfortunately they do not know how the real length is measured. Some men are under such a strong pressure to perform that they consult a physician to get a surgical penis enlargement.

The length of a penis was determined in a study. The men pulled their penis at the glans as long as possible and the centimetres starting at the bony onset (symphysis) up to the external urethra opening were measured. The average penis length was 12.8 cm. Do you still think that your penis is too short? Using this method the lengths were between 10-18 cm. No connection between a person's height and his penis' length was found. Furthermore, there is no relation between potency and the size of the penis. Furthermore, it was found out by questioning the women, that for most of them sexual satisfaction did not depend on the penis size of their sexual partner. There were only a few female exemptions that only can get a sexual climax if the partner has a big penis. But then again there are also men who can only get an orgasm if the partner wears "high heels".

The length of the penis varies greatly and no conclusions to the virility can be made. It is of no importance for a harmonic sexual life how long the penis is. The wish to have a penis-enlargement that many men have, is not a wish of their partner but often comes from the self-made pressure to perform which is widely spread in our society that lives by the motto: "faster, higher, stronger".

Only seldom, in cases of malformations of the genitals, a surgery of the penis is performed.

We men should keep in mind that it is not the length of the penis that is important but how we use it.

3.2.2 Fear of One's Own Sexuality

Many men are restrained or feel guilty about doing or wishing something that they lust for. This means the open and honest handling of one's own sexuality, not extraordinary sexual practises. Often the reason for getting this bad conscience is something acquired in childhood from the parents or the society. Some older couples have never seen their partner naked during full daylight and although they have been married for many years, they only have sex in the darkness. The older generation here has a disadvantage to the younger one since the younger one learns to be much more open about sexuality.

An excessive sense of shame makes it difficult or even impossible to speak about sexual wishes or act with according devotion. This mental conflict between the inner needs and the external surroundings can cause men to suffer from impotency and women to have trouble with orgasms.

3.2.3 Sexuality Under Pressure to Perform and Fear to Fail

The pressure to perform is very strong in today's society, we all want to be successful with regard to our jobs and private lives. Expectations born from the society or the partner can be the reason for sexual problems. The media show the picture of a man that is always successful and always ready for sex, too. Similar symptoms to the 1970s, when the ideal of the women's world was a Twiggy-figure which started an era of hysteric diets and many anorexic women, are developing in the men's world now.

Many men do not see the world of feelings, which normally plays a big role, in the sexuality of showing performance at least 2-3 times a week. In the consume-routine the emotional part almost gets left out entirely. Erotic movies and male friends bragging about supposedly numerous sexual acts give us the wrong ideas about performances. If one cannot keep up to the action of the men shown in the movies and the remarks made when men are among each other, one feels like he is not a real man anymore. Sometimes one feels like a loser then. Especially sexually inexperienced men have a totally incorrect picture about what sexuality is all about. It is therefore no surprise that they are very afraid to fail during their first sexual contacts and the pressure is so great that an erection is not possible. Even sexually experienced men can "fail" occasionally if the pressure to perform is too strong. It is also not surprising that the thought of having sex at least weekly – although this amount does not meet with the individual desire to have sex – can lead to the case that neither body nor soul is willing to produce the performance suggested.

This often results in frustrating attempts to have sex which accordingly lower the man's self-esteem. Afterwards this man will fear not to keep up with the pressure to perform which subsequently results in a continuous "failing" although there is no organic reason for this. There is a misunderstanding between the pressure to keep up with certain socially related performance demands on the one hand and one's own sexual demands and individual physical readiness for performance on the other hand.

The female partner hardly ever places such an exaggerated performance demand onto the man. For women sexuality is much more based on emotions. Exaggerated sexual demands from the partner are very seldom the reason for problems to get an erection.

It hardly ever happens that a woman makes fun of the man or degrades him because of his possible sexual weaknesses. If this is the case, however, it can certainly be the reason for fear of failure in the male and the symptoms for impotence can be caused by it or even strengthened by it.

3.2.4 If One Loses One's Nerves

The process for sexual reactions is controlled and co-ordinated mostly by nerves. Therefore it is not surprising, that even the strongest man suffers from "stage-fright" before the first time with a new partner. The hands get wet, the heart starts beating more strongly, the blood pressure goes up rapidly and you are nervous. These are the same symptoms our ancestors, the hunters, experienced. The only difference is that this was the preparation of their body to be ready for the coming fight or the escape in order to produce maximum performance and not to become sexually active and to have sex to reproduce. During the fight and escape situation the life of the man was in danger and his strengths were fully concentrating on the approaching action. Nobody expected reactions of the penis in these situations. These were situations of life and death. Therefore it is no surprise that during these tense physical reactions – not only for our ancestors and not only for hunters, there was no erection.

3.3 Organic (Physical) Causes

New methods of examinations have been developed which make it possible for patients who suffer from erectile dysfunction, meaning disturbances in the ability to get erections over a prolonged period of time, to get a detailed diagnosis for the cause of this malfunction.

Organic factors are the cause in 55-85% of the cases suffering from erection problems. In approximately 25-35% of these cases the mental factor also plays an important role. If it is physically impossible to have sex over a longer period of time, often there is the additional side effect of suffering psychological disturbances as well. This is also the case when the problems that are causing the erectile dysfunction to begin with are of a purely physical nature.

We distinguish between different organic causes that can be the cause of impotence.

3.3.1 Problems with the Blood Supply

Problems with the blood supply often are the cause of an organically caused impotence. Either this problem is caused by hereditary malformations of the vessels or it is an acquired disturbance of the blood circulation, the latter being more common. The reason for the primary impotence of a male that becomes sexually active for the first time can for example be the absence of the supplying vessels (arteries) or a malformation (hypoplasy) of the penis arteries. More often so the cause is acquired problems with the blood circulation. This lack of blood supply leads to according deficiency symptoms in the body parts concerned.

Chronic vascular occlusions are to be distinguished from acute ones. Acute vascular occlusions are especially known around the heart. When a clogging of the blood vessel that is the only support of a certain heart muscle region occurs, the myocardial cells go dead after a certain time and the performance of this organ decreases.

Much more often than the acute, the slow (chronic) clogging occurs. In this case usually the inside of the cell gets tighter slowly but continuously due to calcium deposits until the vessel is clogged and no blood can flow through it at all anymore. The calcium deposits in the walls of the vessel are called arteriosclerosis. Arteriosclerosis is a disease that often affects the vascular system of the whole body. It can manifest itself at the heart as angina pectoris (continuously appearing heartache when under physical or mental strain). In the brain increasing disturbances of memory or even temporary lasting symptoms including loss of speech can occur.

The so called window-shopping disease (claudicatio intermittens) which forces the people affected to keep interrupting their walk because of strong pain in the calf or in the thigh, is a result of arteriosclerosis. If the vessel gets totally clogged due to the calcium deposits the person can suffer a heart attack or a stroke and the amputation of the leg might even be necessary – depending on the location of the vessel-clogging. Arteriosclerosis can also occur in the vessel responsible for the penis. It is not well known that general arterioslerotic changes of the vessel can sometimes effect the pelvic and penis vessels first. For only insignificant tightening of the supporting penis arteries can have the effect of not supplying enough blood necessary for an erection. The first sign of an insufficient blood supply manifested in this organ is an erectile dysfunction.

A study was performed in the United States in which all men suffering from difficult problems in getting an erection, had their blood pressure measured by their urologists. This is something that actually should be done on a routine basis when suffering from these problems. All men who were diagnosed with strong circulation problems in their penis then got a entire body check-up with a heart specialist (cardiologist).

The result of this was that 16% of all men suffering from sclerosis of the pelvic or penis arteries had according changes of their heart vessels. Without knowing it, these men were at a high risk to suffer a heart attack. Therefore impotence in some cases can be the first sign of an upcoming heart attack. It is time to rapidly start preventing medical measures to avoid this from happening!

In the following paragraphs the risk factors of arteriosclerosis are briefly talked about.

Smoking

With chronic smokers one talks about a "smoker's leg". Here due to a high consumption of cigarettes a clogging of the vessels in the leg is caused which can eventually lead to a loss of the leg.

Analogous to the "smoker's leg" it would be possible to talk about a "smoker's penis". The increased misuse of nicotine can cause changes of the vessels and lead to impotence.

Smoking does not only seem to have a negative effect on the blood supply but also seems to damage the venous obstructive mechanism. The increased blood-flow out of the penis additionally hinders the stiffening of the penis.

Overweight (Adipositas)

This can lead to a high blood pressure. The blood-fat levels of obese people usually are high and this promotes arteriosclerosis.

High Blood Pressure (Hypertony)

This is a first ranking disease of civilisation with all its negative effects onto the inner radius of the vessels. A damage of the vessel-wall is a long-term result that later on can lead to a lowering of the blood supply of the organ concerned, for example the penis.

Taking medication to lower the blood pressure also can have negative effects on potency.

Diabetes (Diabetes Mellitus)

People suffering from this disease often have calcium deposits on the walls of the vessels (angiopathy), which can manifest in all organs. Especially people with diabetes who are not medically adjusted right, suffer from this problem with the changes of the vessels in a rather short time. Often this leads to damages of the eyes, the kidneys, the heart and the legs, but the penis does not get spared from these negatives effects either. More than 50% of all diabetics are suffering from impotence during the course of their life. Diabetes does not only harm the vessels of the penis but also the neutral paths (polyneuropathy). We have already heard that the function of the nerves has a significant meaning for the process of the erection. If there are misleads or malfunctions of the nerve impulses, an erection might not be possible.

Elevated Blood Fat (Cholesterol, Triglycerid)

Everybody knows that elevated cholesterol levels promote calcification of the vessels. Changes of the vascular structure certainly can also have a negative influence on potency. The elevated cholesterol levels often are caused from a malnutrition or overnutrition, but in a few cases they are due to hereditary problems.

If one or more of the above mentioned risk factors exist, one should know that the possibility to get an erection is at risk on a long-term basis. In this case you should definitely try to change your way of living.

3.3.2 Disturbances of the Venous Blood-flow

A full erection that is needed to have sex can only be accomplished if the blood does not flow out of the penis. The outgoing blood vessels are pressed close when the penis starts getting bigger so less blood can flow out of the cavernous bodies. Because more and more blood is kept in the penis, it stiffens. A sufficient stiffness of the penis is necessary to be able to enter the vagina. The venous back-flow can be increased by the outgoing blood vessels or a disturbed function of the cavernous bodies.

Now it can happen that a sufficient amount of blood flows into the penis and it increases its size (tumescence) but that the stiffness itself that is necessary to penetrate the vagina only is there for a short time or not at all. The normal reduction of the outflow of blood is not there anymore. The blood that is being pumped into the cavernous body remains there only for a short time and quickly flows out again. Here one can also distinguish between hereditary disorders and acquired ones. A primary impotence can be caused by a hereditary leak (cavernous insufficiency) in the cavernous body. Nevertheless these vessel deformities are very seldom. More common are the acquired venous leaks. Due to a lack of elasticity of the cavernous body, the compression of the vessels for the outgoing blood is not sufficient anymore.

Presumably a long-term lack of oxygen supply of the penis leads to a lack of the elasticity of the cavernous body. Therefore changes of the vessels in which they get narrow often exist. The lack of blood circulation can lead to malnutrition of oxygen and nutrients in the cavernous bodies.

This then causes changes inside the penis that finally lead to hardening (sclerosis) and a lack of elasticity of the tissue of the cavernous bodies. In extreme cases a total change of the structure of the cavernous body can be the result. The small honeycombed hollow-rooms are totally inflexible then and can not take up any blood. The cavernous body loses its elasticity and cannot unfold itself anymore. When palpating it, it feels hard even when not erected. Due to the hardening of the cavernous body it is not possible anymore for the penis to fill with blood and extend even when being sexually stimulated.

Another cause for the increased outflow of blood could be the formation of a new vein and the incapacity of the out-flowing vessels to narrow their transverse section. Using special examinations, the urologist can find out whether a general venous back-flow of the blood is there or whether a certain vessel is not able to lower the back-flow of blood sufficiently.

3.3.3 Disorder of the Nerves (Neurological Reasons)

Some neurological disorders can cause a sexual dysfunction. On the one hand this can be a defect (caused by an accident or surgery) of the peripheral nerve system which disturbs the impulses coming from or going to the genital organs making it impossible to transmit information to or from the superior nerve bundle of the pelvis, the spinal cord or the brain. On the other hand there are a lot of sicknesses that damage the nerve system especially in the spinal cord. Also accidents and injuries of the brain, the spinal cord or nerves can be the reason for impotence.

3.3.4 Hormonal Disorders and Their Cause

The different synergies and triggering hormonal mechanisms are very complex. Contrary to most mammals the human being does not have a season of heat that is driven by hormones. But the corresponding influences on the sex drive (libido) play an important role.

The following groups of hormones influence the sexual behaviour of the human:

■ Androgens are the male sexual hormones; especially testosterone must be mentioned.
■ Oestrogen, for example estradiol, are some of the female sex hormones
■ Prolactin is produced in the pituitary gland
■ Gestagens like progesterone (pregnancy hormone) influence the hormonal status as higher switched mediators

The concentration of hormonal groups differs by gender. In men the androgens are rather dominating, in women the estrogens. The male hormones are mainly produced in the testicles (Leydig cells). In addition, less than 1/10 of androgens are produced in the adrenal gland. Complex control-circles located in certain parts of the brain and in the pituitary gland make sure that there is a hormonal balance.

Lack of testosterone plays a special role in the sexual behaviour, as also does an overproduction of the hormone prolactin (hyperprolactinemia).

Other hormonal disorders, for example over- or underproduction of the thyroid gland, can have an influence on the ability to get an erection.

Finally one should not forget to mention hormones responsible for the sense of smelling (pheromones) that also seem to have an influence on sexual behaviour.

3.3.5 Medical Side-effects

Some medication can cause disorders of erection, ejaculation and libido. Due to their illness most patients need to continue taking these medications. Most of the time these illnesses that need treatment already include the risk of causing problems with the erection. Especially medication for the blood pressure, diabetes, bronchitis and arteriosclerosis should be mentioned here. The treating physician should be informed about newly arising problems with potency so it can be determined individually if it is possible to switch to alternative medication that will not have negative influence on potency.

3.4 Problems with Ejaculation

There are three forms of ejaculation problems: the premature ejaculation (ejaculatio praecox), the unnaturally delayed ejaculation (ejaculatio retardata) and the orgasm without ejaculation (retrograde ejaculation). These different malfunctions are briefly mentioned below:

3.4.1 Premature Ejaculation (Ejaculatio Praecox)

Together with the erectile dysfunction (inability to get an erection) this malfunction is the most common male sexual disorder. With a few exceptions, it is almost always due to psychogenic reasons. When suffering from ejaculatio praecox, sexual intercourse sometimes only lasts a few seconds. After the penetration the ejaculation comes immediately or within a short time frame, causing a slackness of the penis that hinders the continuation of the sexual intercourse. We talk about a premature ejaculation if the ejaculation cannot be held long enough for the partner to be satisfied in at least half of the times when having sexual intercourse.

This is a very vague interpretation making clear that it is not easy to give an exact definition of this condition. Furthermore one should take into consideration that it is in the nature of things to pass the male inheritance onto as many females as possible, for the original sense of cohabitation (sexual intercourse) was only the reproduction and the passing on of the inheritance with it. In times of permanent waiting danger from beast or prey it made sense to pass on the inheritance as quickly as possible. Only due to today's civilised lifestyle the ability to get a fast ejaculation has lost its (high) ranking in the fight to survive and other criterion like the satisfaction of the partner are put first now.

Nowadays ejaculatio praecox can be the cause of significant problems within a relationship. If not treated, it can even lead to giving up any sexual activity at all or in the worst scenario to a separation. Unfortunately even fewer of the men concerned consult a physician than those with an erectile dysfunction do. The emphasis is put on "unfortunately" because by means of behaviour therapy and targeted training and certain exercises as they are explained in the book, the problem can be handled well after a certain time.

3.4.2 Delayed Ejaculation (Ejaculatio Retardata)

This disorder is very seldom and many men dream about having such a disorder. After penetration the time-span to the orgasm and the ejaculation is so long that most women consider it as painful and not lustful. For the men who suffer from this disorder the sexual intercourse often is not too satisfying, either, because they would love to get the "liberating" ejaculation. Often this problem is caused by nerve damages in the ejaculation centre or in the nerves that connect the centre and the penis. But also mental problems and certain medication can have the delay of the ejaculation as a side effect.

3.4.3 Inability to Have an Ejaculation (Retrograde Ejaculation)

In the vernacular this disorder also is called a "dry orgasm". Here the semen is not catapulted into the urethra during the orgasm – but goes backward - (retrograde) – into the bladder and is discharged when urinating at a later point in time. There are different reasons for such a disorder. It could be damage to the peripheral nerve due to increased consumption of alcohol, badly adjusted diabetes or surgery in the stomach or pelvic region, which have caused damage to the network of the nerves. But also changes of the nerves in the ejaculation centre can be the cause for this. A retrograde ejaculation can also be the result of prostate or bladder neck surgeries.

It is of no importance here whether the surgery was performed through the urethra or whether the prostate was removed using an hypogastric cut. Both surgeries almost always destroy the closing mechanism of the neck of the bladder that hinder the semen to get into the bladder during the ejaculation and therefore points into the forward direction out through the urethra.

4 How a Man Can and Should Exercise Potency

4.1 Why Should I Exercise Potency?

The answer is simple: To have a satisfying sex life in all stages of life!

How can you imagine the success you get through this exercise? Let us compare having sexual intercourse with a 3 km run. The athlete who wants to accomplish a good performance on this distance needs a well-balanced training, for example runs of 10 km, 1 km speed runs and 400 metres interval training.

This training makes a lot more sense to get a good result on a 3 km run than monotonously running a distance of 3 kilometres on a regular basis. With potency it is more or less the same.

Instead of regularly having sexual intercourse with your partner – something that is not always possible due to different reasons, you should – just like with the 3 kilometres run – not always run the same distance, but instead exercises around the set goal. In this case you are able to do this with the exercises and training program which are described in this book. Also not everyone is able to run 3 kilometres without taking a break but must exercise to accomplish this performance. Analogous to this you can imagine how potency is functioning.

In the media but also in medical research, more and more talks are about the "male menopause" (climacterium virile) and its sexuality. The male menopause is less of a burden than that of women. 40-50 year old males on average have sex 4-5 times a month, 50-60 year old males about 3 times a month. 25% of the men questioned in this age group said that they do not have sexual intercourse at all anymore, this was caused rather by the inability to get an erection for the lust was still there. Recent inquiries have found out that half of all 70 year old males still have sexual intercourse and an even higher part was still interested in having sex.

39

Naturally the frequency of spontaneous erections gets less when getting older and a secondary erectile dysfunction (although originally it was possible to get good erections, this is no longer the case now) happens more often. The change of the vessels – naturally the blood does not flow as well in older vessels – and the loss of elasticity in the cavernous bodies strongly adds to this problem from an organic point of view. Furthermore the hormone level drops and the libido also shows a decreasing tendency. The time frame needed to get a full erection often is longer when the person is older. The maximum stiffness of the penis is not present anymore.

Men who do not have sex over a longer period of time often have problems in getting an erection. The physical performance capacity and with it the potency should be exercised regularly to keep it or at least delay the loss of it. Viagra has caused its victims! Some of the men who had not been sexually or physically active for a long time before taking the "blue wonder pill" have died after taking it. They just were not exercised enough to meet a new physical "endurance" in their life. A targeted physical training which prepares the man for the pleasant endurance coming up would have been better than just taking the "blue diamond" and suddenly be able to produce top-level performance without being trained.

It therefore is well worth it to keep your "manly vigour" with the help of **VigorRobic®** and even increase it.

4.2 Can Potency Really Be Trained?

If we define "potency" as the ability to be able to have sexual intercourse in a way that should be satisfying for the partner as well, the question definitely can be answered with "yes".

It is possible to exercise
- an increase of the blood circulation, which is combined with a better or increased oxygen support of the penis, as well as
- limit the amount of blood flowing out of the erected penis as well as
- postponement of the ejaculation and with it prolonging the sexual act.

4.2.1 What You Should Know About It

The mechanism of the erection is strongly influenced by the blood supply of the penis. If no blood flows into the penis, it is not possible for it to fill with blood and become erect. An important factor for the blood supply is the ability of the blood vessels (arteries) to supply blood. Once the blood is inside the penis, the mechanisms have to be activated which "hold" the blood in the cavernous bodies. This means that the outflow of blood (venous outflow) is lowered. Both together, the circulation of the penis and the decreased outflow of blood is necessary to get an erection. It is also important that the tissue of the penis is able to extend. It has to be extendable in order to take in the blood volume flowing new into the penis.

In order to exercise potency efficiently, one at first has to understand the meaning of the mechanism for erection and a sufficient oxygen support for being able to get an erection. Later on you will find out how to use this knowledge for the correct exercises and an adequate training program.

Increasing the Oxygen Supply

We know that during the limp phase the blood in the penis does not have a lot of oxygen in it.

During the erection, the oxygen pressure in the penis increases to 3-4 times of the level when resting. There is a connection between the smooth muscular system, the elastic tissue and the honeycomb-like structure. The development and the ratio of the mentioned structures inside the penis are influenced by the oxygen supply.

A long-term good oxygen supply of the penis is supposed to prevent a hardening of the tissue (IPP: induratio penis plastica). IPP is as common as diabetes, therefore it is a disorder one should pay attention to. The older the examined male population, the more often small hard knots are found on the penis. These little knots can cause a curvature of the penis when erected because the tissue can not extend without problems during the phase when it is filled with blood. Sexual intercourse can be painful for both partners due to this curvature. It can also be so pronounced that it will not be possible to penetrate the curved erected penis into the vagina. A good oxygen supply of the cavernous bodies seems to prevent such a disorder with all its unpleasantness.

While sleeping, each man has an average of 3-5 erections. Now the question is raised: Why did nature provide men with this ability? Which biological mechanism and processes are started by these nightly erections? These automatic erections which are there in $1-1^1/_2$-hour intervals while sleeping cause an additional circulation of the outer genitalia. The increased blood circulation causes an increased oxygen pressure in the penis. Getting this oxygen supply is a preventive measure in regard to unnatural hardening (fibrosis), for example nodules building in the penis. Metabolism activities are started which are necessary to keep the balance between the different structures. Concisely spoken, these increases of blood supply do not only seem to keep the tissue of the penis flexible by supporting the elastic structure with sufficient oxygen, but also provide a good ability to get an erection as well.

The question is raised now whether biochemical and physiological processes also depend on the oxygen supply. Normally the oxygen pressure in the limp penis is the same as in the veins (outgoing pathways of used blood). Under these circumstances of decreased oxygen supply, nitrogen monoxide (NO) in the cavernous bodies is not produced. And what does that mean? You might think that you do not need nitrogen monoxide anyway. That is a harmful gas. – Far from it! NO is one of the most important substances necessary to get an erection! Without NO nothing happens at all! If there were no NO the smooth muscles would not slacken (relaxation). And if these muscles do not slacken, the honeycomb hollow-rooms cannot be filled with blood. The result: No erection.

In addition it was found out that the smooth muscles in the penis do not react as well to NO if the oxygen supply is lower. For the production of NO in the body the activity of a certain enzyme (a mediator that leads one substance into another) is very important. This enzyme seems to need an increased oxygen concentration in order to work better or to work at all. Therefore we can come to the conclusion that a good oxygen supply of the cavernous body is very important to have a satisfying sex life.

For men who have a lower blood supply of their penis because the supplying vessels are constricted or clogged, erections are hard to get or not possible at all because the supplying vessels going to the penis cannot increase the blood-flow in the penis and with it the concentration of oxygen that is necessary.

Last but not least, it should be mentioned that even medication cannot help to get an erection if the oxygen concentration of the cavernous bodies is too low.

Just how important the oxygen supply of the penis is for an erection, became apparent with patients suffering from a chronic obstructive (clogged) pulmonary disease. If the oxygen supply was increased for patients suffering from the symptoms of erectile dysfunction, they were able to get an erection again.

Increasing the Blood Supply

It was found out that regular erections are able to influence the ability to stay potent. Not only the metabolism processes are important which need an increased oxygen demand but also the vessels that supply the oxygen have to bring a certain performance. You have just found out that in the filling phase of the erection the radius of the blood vessels transporting the oxygen significantly increases and the speed of the blood is increased many times over. This process however can only be accomplished in healthy, vessels that are "in good shape".

In order to be able to keep your ability to get an erection, a regular usage of the blood supplying vessels is necessary. The vessels of the pelvis as well as those of the penis have to be subject to different rates of blood supply/flow. First of all to prepare the vessels for the endurance caused by an increased blood flow and secondly to enable an additional vascularization (angiogenesis).

Unfortunately the elasticity of the vessels decreases when getting older. Often calcium deposits built on the walls of the vessels that can cause calcification up to a vascular occlusion. A regular increase of the blood flow has the effect of a better nutrient supply as well as a prevention of calcium deposits on the walls that will guarantee a good circulation in the future.

Lowering the Outflow of Blood

All of the muscles in the pelvic diaphragm, the perineal ischiocavernosus (IC) and bulbospongiosus (BS) muscles included, are activated while having sexual intercourse and therefore cause a higher pressure in the erected penis. Due to these muscle activities and due to the filling of the honeycomb-like hollow room structures with blood to the maximum, the resistance of the blood vessels for the outgoing blood is increased by approximately 100 times. This increase of pressure is necessary to have sexual intercourse.

Impotent patients who suffer from an increased outflow of blood from the penis are tried to be helped by a surgery that logically tries to prevent the high outflow. If too much blood flows out of the penis, the outflow simply should be slowed down – this way the blood stays in the penis for a longer duration. But who likes the idea of getting some veins cut to lower the outflow of blood out of the penis? Are there any other possibilities as well? Yes, a ring that is applied on the outside and which compresses the outgoing blood vessels so strongly that less blood can flow out of the penis. These rings are for sale in different variations and can also be subscribed by a physician if there are certain indications for it.

What other methods are there to reduce the outflow of the blood? – Your own muscles! The stiffness and hardness of the penis can be improved by a targeted training! A group of patients suffering from increased outflow of blood regularly exercised a certain program for four months. Afterwards it was possible for most of the patients to reach an increase of stiffness by an average of 24% in the base of the penis and of about 31% at the point of it. With an increased penis pressure like this it was possible again to penetrate into the vagina. At the same time the electric activities of the IC muscles were measured. The data showed an increased activity of the IC muscles when the penis pressure was randomly increased. Flexing the IC muscle especially had a positive influence on the stiffness of the penis, especially the point of it.

Those men who have problems to penetrate into the vagina at the first sexual contact often will be able to overcome these problems with the help of targeted training. Also for men who are not able to build up enough hardness in the penis after they have already had an orgasm, it will be possible to have sexual intercourse more often after exercising for a certain time. We know that when getting older the stiffness of the penis gets less. When exercising regularly, this effect can be delayed or even prevented. Further studies have shown that not only the stiffness of the penis can be improved by activating the IC and BC muscles, but the outflow of blood in the penis clearly can be reduced as well, causing an increase of pressure in the penis. If more blood is led into a room which cannot extend any more, this increases the inside pressure. For the penis this means maximum stiffening.

Delaying the Ejaculation
The muscles that will be trained by the later described exercises, are a part of the control of the "ejaculation reflex". Men suffering from early ejaculations can delay these with the help of targeted training of the pelvic diaphragm. Men who are not satisfied with the duration of their erection can also learn to control the "ejaculation reflex" by targeted training. By delaying the ejaculation, the duration of stiffness of the penis can be prolonged. This way you can bring yourself and your partner more joy with the newly learned "endurance". But please do not train for a marathon! Your partner then could suffer from pain in the vagina and experience discomfort.

Think about this: With the help of a targeted training the perineal muscles, the IC and BS muscles you can delay your ejaculation and with this exercise a prolongation of the sexual intercourse!

4.3 Who Is Suitable for this Training?

The Urological-andrological Point of View

Under the following conditions a successful training is possible:
The hormone parameter (testosterone, prolactin, FSH and LH) shows a normal level. The supplying blood vessels (arteries) of the penis show no

pathological (unhealthy) changes. There is no increased outflow of blood from the penis during the erection. There are regular, normal nightly erections.

With according medical machines the values can be recorded.

If one of the above mentioned parameters is not in accordance with the norm or if there is a strong psychological component, this can influence the desired training success. Certainly healthy men get the best results when doing **VigorRobic®**.

Physical (Cardiovascular-orthopaedic) Point of View

In principal, all men 16 years or older can start **VigorRobic®**. If there are any symptoms of a disorder, only a part of the training program should be performed. A physician will give you further information on this. If suffering from irregularity of pulse, extrasystoles or general cardiovascular diseases (this also includes elevated blood pressure), if you have back, spinal or joint problems or if you were admitted to the hospital or had surgery within the last years as well as when feeling sick, you should at any case consult a physician before you start exercising.

It is better to contact a physician one time too many than not enough. Starting at the age of 35, everybody should get a physical check-up every two years. And do not forget to regularly get a check-up with a urologist starting at the age of 40. Make sure to go by the suggestion of the health insurance – precaution is better than to have all one's trouble for nothing.

5 Basic Rules of Vigor*Robic*®- Training

It is important to cautiously start with **Vigor*Robic*®** especially if you have worked-out only little or not at all before. This suggestion also is valid if you have had a longer training pause. Once the first progress is visible often this leads to only doing the exercises which have been easy to do from the beginning. Do not follow this inner desire! Even if you have problems to follow the motions as they are shown in the exercises at first, do not give up and keep in mind that just the effort of trying is training itself already! After a certain time I am sure you will be able to do the exercises. Especially because the exercises which are harder to do take more effort from you, you should practise them more often. If it is possible, you should have your motions controlled by an expert from time to time. This is to prevent the wrong movements from sneaking in.

Do not forget to warm-up well before every training unit. One more important advice: Listen to warning signs of your body!

If you want to train the stableness of the erection in the same training unit as the increase of blood circulation it is important to at first exercise the muscles that are responsible for slowing down the outflow of blood. After that a program to increase the penile blood circulation should follow. Why should you keep this order? Even afterwards the training for the improvement of the oxygen support of the penis causes a better circulation in the penis. This advantage would be decreased if putting the exercises in a reverse order because the flexing of muscles reduces the circulation in smaller blood vessels.

5.1 Warm-up and Cooling Down

The training program consists of three phases: Warm-up, training, and cooling down. With the warm-up you are preparing the body for the training. The rise in temperature in the muscle makes it possible to contract (pull itself together, work) with more strength enabling a more intensive training. If the body temperature rises, certain metabolism processes work more effectively. The heart rate rises, the circulation of blood increases, the respiration is more intensive and the waste not needed in the metabolism (slag) can more easily be discharged. The warm-up lowers the risk to get injured, for example spraining or straining.

More synovial fluid is produced in the joint cavity. An easy run or a moderate aerobic- or gymnastic-like warm-up is recommended.
If you plan on working out with weights, you should at first exercise using a low weight and a high amount of repetitions. With these easy warm-up sets you are preparing the muscles, tendons and joints for the increase in resistance.

You will know by a light film of sweat building on your skin and the freshening of our facial colour that the warm-up is right and the exercises are not too low in their intensity. Keep in mind: The warm-up is supposed to be preparing and motivating, not exhausting and frustrating.
The duration of the warm-up program does not only depend on the type of warm-up, which you can choose individually, it also depends on the time of the day and the temperature. You should warm-up longer and more carefully in the mornings than you need to in the evenings. The same is valid if the temperature is low.

After completing the training a cool down phase follows. This means: You slowly start the training program and finish-up as slow. The cardiovascular system slowly goes back to its original unencumbered condition. The metabolism of the muscles eases and the mind relaxes. Just like with the warm-up phase you can use different forms of cooling down as well.

5.2 Frequency of Training

A long-lasting improvement and conservation of the "current" shape you are in can only be accomplished when training regularly. You should try to do the exercises for the stableness and the training program to improve the blood circulation at least 2-3 times a week. You can also combine both goals set in the training if you do exercises for the training of the steadiness after the warm-up and afterwards those to improve your blood circulation. The training should be accomplished at least twice a week. Nevertheless one training unit is better than none at all.

The exercises and training units are very intensive; therefore you should always take a break in between the training units of one group. Certainly you can also train six times a week, for example Monday, Wednesday and Friday exercises to improve the stableness and Tuesday, Thursday and Saturday exercises to improve the circulation. After such a strenuous week it is no problem to take a break from exercising on Sundays.

5.3 Individual Performance Limits

Each individual has a different exercise tolerance and an individual performance capacity. If you have not been doing any sports for a longer duration of time, you should carefully start your training. Regular training will enable you to increase your potency and maintain the level you are used to for years. Especially sexually inactive men notice a loss of capacity after having been sexually inactive for a longer period of time.

Prevent this from happening by keeping your penis "fit" with other activities during these periods of life. Keep up or improve your quality of life. But start slowly and use the right dosage of training. Keep in mind: You have all the time in the world!

5.4 Warning Signals of the Body

Listen to the signals your body is sending you! If you feel pain or other signs of overuse, you should consult a physician and get a check-up. Muscle soreness often comes if you are not used to moving a lot and through strenuous activities. Relax! Take a hot bath or do the exercises of the next training unit at a lower pace to accelerate the process of regeneration. The sore muscles are normally caused by microscopically small injuries. After two to three days these symptoms will have disappeared again.

And once again the advice: When suffering from chills and fever, a cold or acute signs of having an infection you should pause with the training even when you are highly motivated. Bad damages like lung inflammations and inflammation of the myocardium can be caused if you ignore these signals. This can lead to conditions that will restrict your quality of life up to life-threatening situations.

5.5 Performance Decrement Due to Over-exercising

I understand well that you want to be successful within a short time and it is really good to be motivated. If you cannot measure up to this new physical demand, a training that is performed too often or too intensively can even lead to a performance decrement. Therefore you should slowly increase the intensity and the volume of the training! A sign of overtraining can sometimes be muscle and joint soreness. Another one that points towards this is constant tiredness and weariness. If this is the case, you have not given your body enough time to recover. Do not be surprised that this can lead to a lasting performance decrement, dullness and laziness.

So, do not develop the wrong kind of ambition, this has often caused quite the opposite! Set yourself realistic goals and get to the training using your presence of mind!

5.6 Get to Know the Body

It is recommended to concentrate on certain parts of the body, this way you get to know your body better and understand how the different motions work together with the muscles. Especially at the beginning it is important to relax and develop a good feeling about your body. You have to learn to listen to your body. Try to feel the muscle you are training right now in the way it works and try to imagine the individual groups of muscles working together. Start cautiously and slowly increase the amount of repetitions. Every individual is different.

For some **VigorRobic®** is very easy, it is also a matter of how well trained you are already. Others will need a longer approach time until they will be able to effectively use the exercises to experience the success.

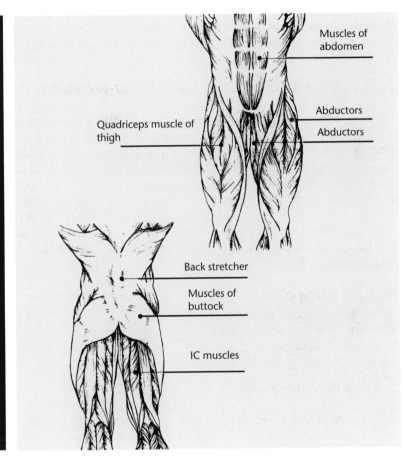

Figure 6: Muscles to get acquainted with

First of all get to know the anatomy of your body. Find out where the muscles are that you want to train. Develop a feeling for the muscles and learn to differentiate between the different groups of muscles like the abdomen, buttocks, back of femora (IC muscles), front of femora, adductor, abductor (figure VI) and the pelvic diaphragm, especially of the BS and IC muscles. Do not be too shy to touch the muscles to feel the activation and change of them during training. Simply put your hands on the different muscles.

It is especially important, to feel the pelvic diaphragm and the BS and IC muscles. To do so, put two fingers in the region between testicle and anus. In most people the fat tissue there is small enough to make it possible to feel the muscles underneath it, especially if you randomly flex them. Even after training for a couple of weeks or months, even after years you should from time to time control the effect and right performance of the exercises by feeling the muscles trained (with the hand).

The BS and IC muscles are flexed by the following exercise: Please take up a standing position. The legs are about shoulder width apart, the points of the feet are slightly turned outwards. Keep your upper body upright. The shoulders are slightly pulled back *(picture 1)*.

Imagine you are holding a coin between the muscles of your buttocks. It would fall down if you would not activate your muscles. Try to put such a strong pressure on the coin as if you would try to "press the incuse together". Now also imagine that a small cloth covers your penis. Try to move the

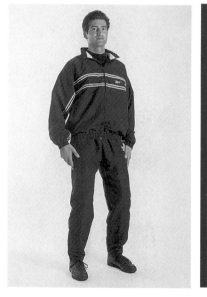

Picture 1

52

cloth in the direction of your belly using the penis. Try harder! Do not forget your breathing and feel the flexed muscles between the testicle and the anus with your fingers *(figure 7)*.

These are the muscles you should train! Intensify this feeling of muscle tension. Now relax and just drop the thought about the cloth and the coin – Certainly these exercises to "feel the body" can also be performed using real things.

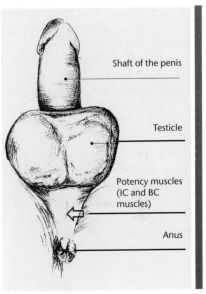

Figure 7: Getting acquainted with the potency muscles

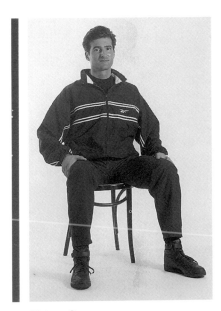

Picture 2

Here a further exercise to get to know the pelvic diaphragm and the BS and IC muscles: Sit down on a chair, the legs are slightly apart. The upper body is held in a straight position *(picture 2)*.

Your upper thighs should make a right angle. Now imagine you would be sitting on a pillow filled with rice (or you can use a 15 x 15 cm big pillow filled with 180 g of rice to do the exercises realistically). Breathe calmly and when inhaling imagine how you "suck" the rice grains upwards

53

with the bottom of the pelvis. Feel how the pelvic diaphragm tightens! At the same time there is a slight pressure on the urethra. You have to memorise this feeling because this is the tension that should be reached during all of the following exercises.

Have fun when getting acquainted with the potency muscles!

PART II – EXERCISES AND TRAINING PROGRAMS

6 Exercises for Maintaining a Steady Erection

When performing the following exercises, it is very important that you listen to your body. Do not force yourself, simply use strength!

■ Try to relax before each training session to mentally prepare yourself for the work-out that is coming up.

■ The movements at first should be light and slow. For the advanced training it is also important to keep a certain basic tension during all of the muscle training.

■ After finishing your training, take at least a couple minutes of time to consciously relax.

A Couple of Hints Beforehand Concerning Movement Execution

Make all movements slowly and controlled, without swinging and jerking. Swinging movements put a high strain on the ligaments, joints and bony structures.

Radius of Movement

The exercises should be performed using the whole movement radius possible for the muscles and joints. Through principle you should know that strength increase and improved endurance of the muscle is only valid for the radius and angle trained during the performance of the exercise.

Training Form

When training you should always start with the easiest version of the exercise. If you master the exact performance of the basic exercise, you can build on that and move on to a more difficult version.

Choosing Your Exercise

Not only exercises that directly effect potency are described below. A one-sided training would lead to an imbalance between the muscles that tend to weaken and those that rather tend to shorten. Such a muscular imbalance would increase the risk to get hurt during training. You do not want to harm your body but instead keep or even increase your potency.

To prevent a muscular imbalance, according strengthening exercises should be added to the program.

6.1 Muscle Exercises Without Devices

1. Pelvic Swing

Purpose: Exercising the pelvic diaphragm, BS, IC muscles and muscles of buttocks, the upper legs get a minimum of training as well.

Starting Position: Stand up straight, the legs are about shoulder-width apart. Bend the knees a little bit. The buttocks are slightly stretched backwards so you make a hollow back *(picture 3)*.

Movement Execution: Tighten the muscles of your buttocks to straighten up the pelvis forwards. Hold this position and tighten the buttocks and the BS and IC muscles even more. Continue to breathe in and out calmly while doing so *(picture 4)* – then you decrease the tightening of the muscles again and bring the pelvis back to the starting position.

Variation: Different foot positions are possible. You can have the feet and the knees close together or have the feet pointing outwards shoulder width apart. In the latter version you should additionally tighten the inside muscles of the upper leg to their maximum when finishing the motion. This pressing together even stimulates the pelvic diaphragm, BS and IC muscles even more.

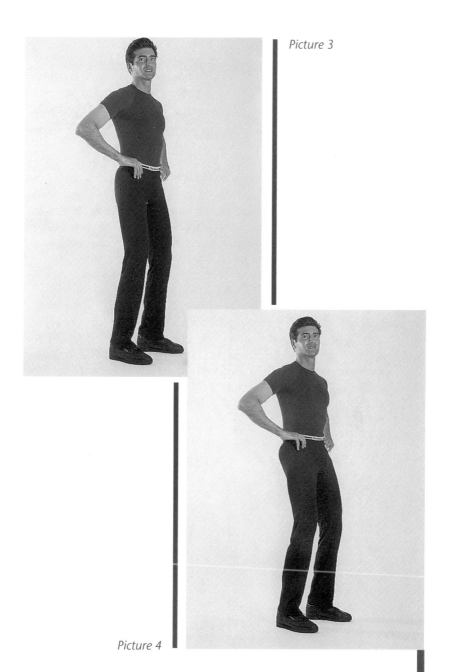

Picture 3

Picture 4

2. Squatting With Pelvic Swing

Purpose: Training the pelvic diaphragm, BS and IC muscles, buttocks and upper leg muscles.

Starting Position: Stand up straight, the legs are shoulder-width apart. Slightly bend your knees. This starting position is the same as in the preceding exercise.

Movement Execution: Increase the knee-bend a little now so the upper legs stay above the horizontal *(picture 5)*. Keep the back straight during this motion. Tighten the muscles of your buttocks to bring the pelvis forward in this position and then straighten it out. Hold this position and tighten the muscles and the BS and IC muscles even more *(picture 6)*. Loosen up and move the pelvis back. Now slowly return to the starting position by straightening out your legs. But not all the way! A certain amount of tension should be kept at all times. Repeat this exercise.

Variation: Here also different foot positions as described in exercise (1) are possible. A further variation is to switch the starting position with the position at the end. This means that you at first would start with a deeper knee-bend. From this position you move upward (starting position of the exercise above). Then a forward tipping of the pelvis follows building-up an increased tension in the muscles that are to be trained. Then loosen up and go back to the starting position. This variation is a little easier but not as effective.

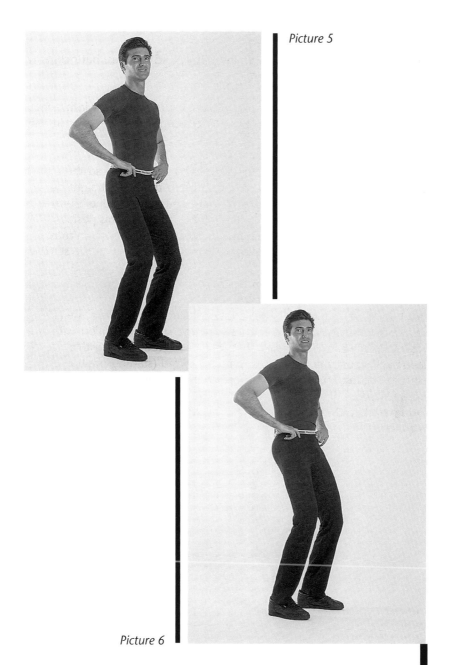

Picture 5

Picture 6

3. Little Pelvic Lift

Purpose: Exercising the pelvic diaphragm, BS and IC muscles, buttocks and ischiocrural muscles (hamstrings) and of the back extensors.

Starting Position: Lie down flat on your back on the ground, the legs bent only sligthly, the point of the feet show upwards and are hip-width apart. The hands are lying on the ground next to the hips *(picture 7)*.

Movement Execution: Tighten the muscles of the buttocks and the back extensors to pick the pelvis up off the ground just a little bit *(picture 8)*. Hold this position and tighten the muscles of the buttocks and the BS and IC muscles even more. Try to breathe in a relaxed manner. Now slowly move back into the starting position and relax. Repeat this motion. During the exercise the feet and shoulders are not moving.

Caution: When suffering from back problems you should consult a physician who should first give his approval for this kind of exercise.

Variation: Once again different foot positions are possible:
1.   Feet and knees are together.
2.   The feet stay about shoulder-width apart.

At the highest point of this motion, the muscles of the inside of the upper legs are additionally flexed to the maximum. This pressing together stimulates the pelvic diaphragm, BS and IC muscles even more.

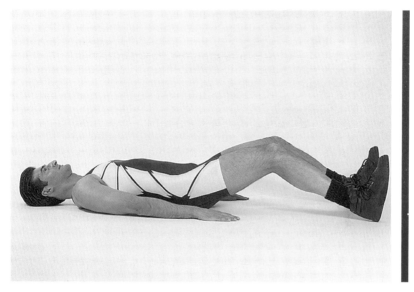

Picture 7

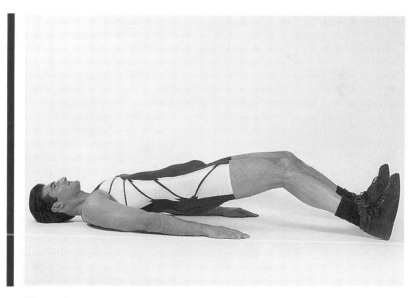

Picture 8

4. Little Pelvic Lift With Leg Lift

Purpose: This is an intensive movement for the pelvic diaphragm, BS and IC muscle, muscles of the buttocks and of the back extensors. Especially the three muscles mentioned at first are getting an intensive training here, more intensive than in the exercise before.

Starting Position: Use the same starting position as in exercise (3). Lie down on the floor flat on your back, the legs are bent only a little bit, the feet are about shoulder-width apart, pointing upwards. The hands are placed on the floor next to the hips.

Movement Execution: Flex the muscles of your buttocks and your back extensors in order to lift the pelvis off the ground. Hold this position at the highest point. Tighten your buttocks and the BS and IC muscles even more. Now slowly move one foot of the almost stretched out leg upward *(picture 9)*. Intensify the tension in the stretched leg by actively flexing the muscles in it. Put the foot back on the floor and slowly return to your

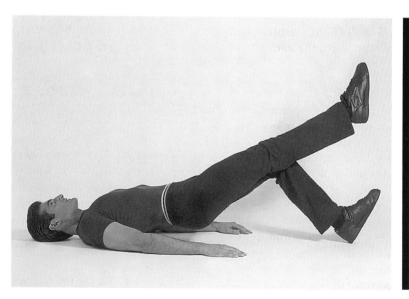

Picture 9

starting position. Repeat this movement. Do not move your feet and shoulders during the entire exercise.

Caution: Also take caution here if you have back problems, the same as mentioned before is valid here. Doing this exercise is more demanding than the one before. Therefore do not be frustrated if it does not work perfect right away.

Variation: You can either take turns lifting a leg in the upper position or first train one side, then the other. To make the exercise more difficult, you can lift one foot off the ground and keep it up from the beginning. If you have finished training one side of your body this way, switch to the other side. The position of the feet can be changed just as in the exercise described before.

5. Pelvic Lift

Purpose: This is a very intensive movement for the pelvic diaphragm, BS and IC muscles, muscles of the buttocks and the back extensors.

Starting Position: Lie on your back, the legs are angled, the feet are hip-width apart, the soles of the feet are flat on the ground, the hands are on the ground next to the hips *(picture 10)*.

Movement Execution: Tighten the muscles of the buttocks and the back extensors to lift the pelvis off the ground. Hold this position at the highest point when the upper legs make one line with the stomach *(picture 11)*. Tighten the muscles of the buttocks as well as the BS and IC muscles even more. Slowly return to your starting position, keeping the buttocks always at one to two finger's widths off the ground. Touch the ground with your buttocks, always keeping the tension in the muscles. Repeat this movement. Feet and shoulders are not moving during the entire exercise.

Caution: If you suffer from back problems consult a physician before doing this exercise.

Variation: For this exercise once again different positions for the feet and knees are possible (as described in 3).

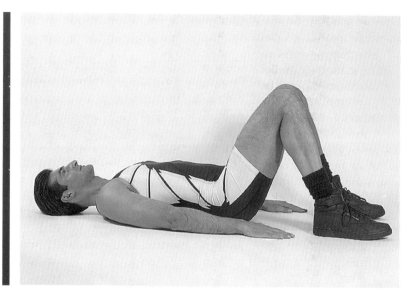

Picture 10

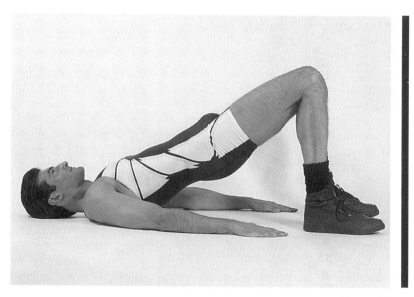

Picture 11

1. Feet and knees are together.
2. If the feet stay shoulder-width apart, you can bring the knees together. This pressing-pressure increases the tension in the IC, BS muscles and pelvic diaphragm. But at the same time the pressure on the knee cap increases. So please be careful with this variation!

While doing this exercise you can spread the knees apart after starting with them together, until you get to the end of the movement. When returning the buttocks to their starting position, you can move the knees together again. The reverse variation is to start the exercise with the knees apart and bring them together during the exercise and bring them apart again when going back to the starting position. By closing the knees in the final position the IC, BS muscles and pelvic diaphragm get the maximum of stimulation.

The distance of the feet to the buttocks can also be changed: If you put your feet close to the pelvis *(picture 11a)*, the muscles of the buttocks are trained more than they are if the knees are only bent slightly: In the latter case more strain is put onto the ischiocrural muscles.

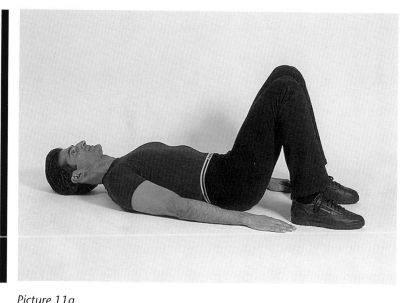

Picture 11a

6. Pelvic Lift With Foot Lift

Purpose: This is a further intensive exercise for the pelvic diaphragm, BS, IC muscles, the muscles of the buttock and the back extensors.

Starting Position: Use the same starting position as in exercise (5). Lie down with the back on the floor, the legs are angled, the feet are hip-width apart, the soles of the feet are flat on the ground, the hands are placed beside the hips on the ground.

Movement Execution: Flex the muscles of your buttocks and your back extensors to lift the pelvis off the ground. Hold this position at its highest point. Flex the muscles of your buttocks as well as the BS and IC muscles even more. Now lift one foot from the ground *(picture 12)*. This increases the tension. Place the foot back onto the ground and slowly return to the starting position, the buttocks should always stay about the width of 2-3 fingers off the ground. Repeat this movement. The feet and shoulders are not moving during the entire exercise.

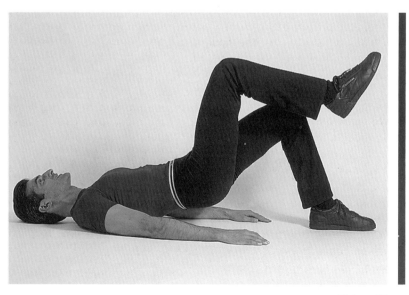

Picture 12

Caution: If you suffer from back problems you should consult a physician.

Variation: You can either take turns lifting the feet to the high position or train one side and then continue with the other. Once you have done training one side of the body, switch to the other. A further possibility is to pick up the right foot when you are in the final position – you increase the tension by doing so - and then put it back down onto the ground. You remain in the final position and now pick up the foot of the other side. You can then – while remaining in the final position – take turns with the side. Finally both feet return to the ground which will bring you back to the starting position.
      You can also vary the distance of the feet to the buttocks during this exercise.

7. Pelvic Lift With Leg Extension

Purpose: This is a very intensive movement for the pelvic diaphragm, BS and IC muscles, muscles of the buttocks and back extensors. Especially the three muscles mentioned at first are trained very intensively here. This one is even more intensive than the exercise before.

Starting Position: The same starting position as in exercise (5) is used. Lie down with your back on the floor, the legs are angled, the feet are hip-width apart, the soles flat on the ground, the knees are together, the hands are on the ground parallel to the hips.

Movement Execution: Lift the pelvis off the ground. Hold this position on its highest point so the upper thighs are making a straight line with the stomach. Flex the buttocks muscles, the BS and IC muscles even more. Now slowly stretch the lower leg until the leg is straightened out all the way *(picture 13)*. Increase the tension in the stretched leg by actively flexing those muscles. In addition, you press the knees together tightly. This is very strenuous! The stretched out leg now is moved back, the knees stay together. Slowly return to the starting position, always keeping the buttocks at least 2 fingers high of the ground, just like in the exercise described above (6). Repeat this movement, feet and shoulders are not moving during this entire exercise.

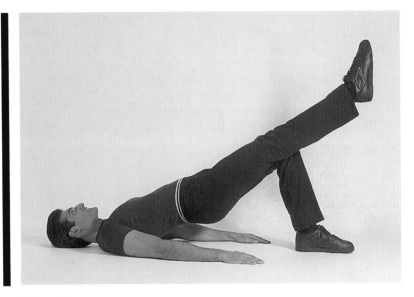

Picture 13

Purpose: This is a very intensive movement for the pelvic diaphragm, BS and IC muscle, muscles of the buttocks and back extensors.

Caution: Here you also should be careful when suffering from back problems and the same advice as mentioned above is valid here, too. The pressure that is put onto the kneecap is not really low, either. If you have knee problems already, make sure to consult a physician for advice before doing this exercise. This exercise is also more demanding than the others.

Variation: You can either switch the legs in the high position, using one after the other or at first exercise one side of the body and then the other. There are two variations for the foot that can be used when the leg is stretched out. You can stretch the foot to a point *(picture 14)* or pull it strongly towards the body (flexing) *(picture 15)*. To make this exercise more effective you can start with a stretched leg from the beginning. It is important that the knees will be pressed together while doing so to build up a maximum pressure for the pelvis.

   The position of the foot as well as the distances can be varied just as in the exercise described before.

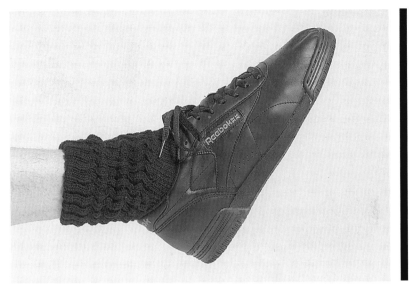

Picture 14

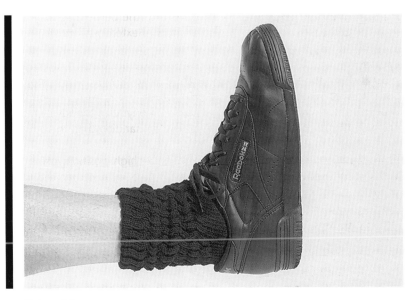

Picture 15

8. Pelvic Lift With Extended Leg

Purpose: The same muscles as in the exercise before (7) are being trained. The tension in the muscles of the buttocks, the pelvic diaphragm and BS and IC muscle is more intensive here.

Starting Position: Lie down with the back on the ground, the legs are angled, the feet are hip-width apart, the soles of the feet flat on the ground, one leg is held up in the air and almost stretched out all the way, the hands are placed on the ground parallel to the hips *(picture 16)*.

Moving Execution: Tighten the muscles of your buttocks and the back extensors to lift the pelvis off the ground. Hold this position at its highest point, the upper thighs are making one line with the stomach *(picture 17)*. Tighten your buttocks muscles and the BS and IC muscles even more. Now slowly return back to the starting position. The buttocks always should stay above the ground about the height of two fingers. Repeat this exercise. Feet and shoulders are not moving during the entire exercise.

Caution: The same precautionary measures are valid as for the exercises before.

Variation: If this exercise is too difficult for you, you can also angle the leg which is in the air more and rest the foot on the knee of the leg which is on the ground *(picture 17a)*. If you want to do this exercise more effectively for the IC and BS muscles then you have to spread out the leg sideways a little (abducted) in the starting position *(picture 17b)*. During the movement back to the final position the leg is moved diagonally above the other *(picture 17c)*. This way the muscles are exercised to the maximum!

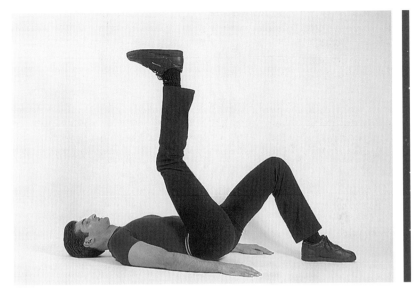

Picture 16

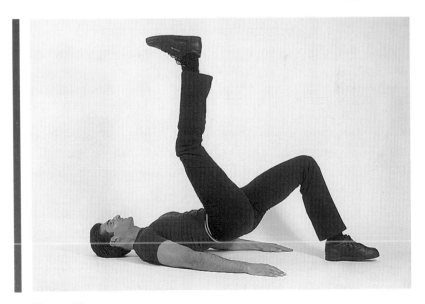

Picture 17

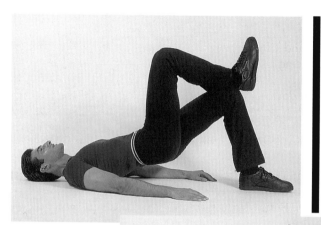

Picture 17a

Picture 17b

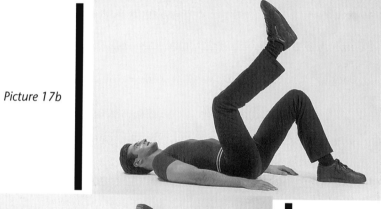

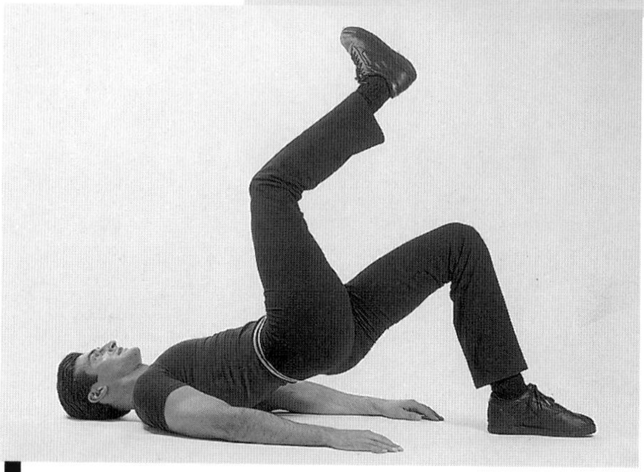

Picture 17c

9. Lifting the Leg from a Prone Position (Boat)

Purpose: The back and buttocks muscles, the pelvic diaphragm, the BS and IC muscles are being trained in this exercise.

Starting Position: Lie down in a prone position, the points of the feet are touching the ground, the legs are stretched out, the feet are hip-width apart, the hands are put under the head so the elbows are pointing outwards *(picture 18)*.

Movement Execution: Tighten the muscles of the buttocks and the back extensors and lift up the stretched out legs a few centimetres off the ground *(picture 19)*. Hold this position and additionally tighten your buttocks muscles, the inside of the upper thighs and the BS and IC muscles even more. Return back to the starting position.

Caution: When suffering from back problems, consult your physician first and get the okay for this exercise. Do not lift up the legs too high because a sway back can develop from that and this can cause damage to the spine.

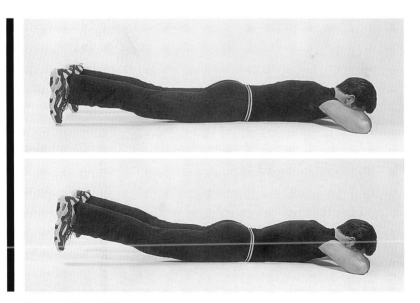

Pictures 18 und 19

Variations: Just as in most of the above mentioned exercises different feet and leg positions are possible here as well. The ankle of the foot and the knee are touching and are lifted upwards in this position. This position makes it a little bit more difficult to tighten the inside of the upper leg. The feet and legs can be spread apart from each other even more than the width of the shoulder. In the upper position it is easier to tighten the adductors then. This causes an additional stimulation to the IC and BS muscles. The feet are flexed in the above mentioned variation (points of feet are pulled towards the shin). Stretching the joints of the feet to their max can build a higher tension in the whole chain of muscles.

10. Scissors in a Prone Position

Purpose: The same as in the above mentioned exercise (9).

Starting Position: Lie down in a prone position again and put your hands under your forehead just as in the above described exercise (9). But now there is a little change in the position of the feet: The points of the feet are pointed backwards so the inner sole of the foot is facing the ground. Lift your legs off the ground as high as possible without making a sway back. Pull the feet apart a little bit now *(picture 20)*.

Movement Execution: Tighten the muscles of your buttocks, the BS and IC muscles when in the position as explained above. Now bring the feet back together crossing one leg a little bit over the other *(picture 21)*. Move the legs apart again and then cross them once more, this time with the other leg on top. Make continuous, slow movements.

Caution: The same precautionary measures are valid here as in the exercise before.

Variations: To make the exercise a little bit easier, you can take turns lifting a stretched out leg with stretched toes. This exercise is more intensive if you stretch out the legs at the same time; this increases the muscle tone. You keep lifting one leg and then switch to the other or simply take turns using the right or left leg.

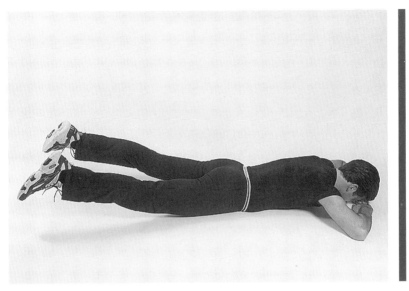

Picture 20

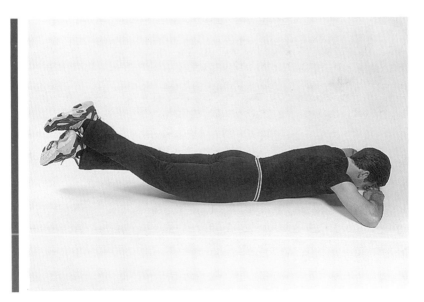

Picture 21

11. Lifting the Trunk from a Prone Position (Cobra)

Purpose: Training of the back extensors and buttocks muscles, the pelvic diaphragm, and the BS and IC muscles.

Starting position: The same starting position is used as in exercise (9). Lie down on your belly, the points of the feet are on the ground, about hip width apart, pointing downwards, the hands are placed underneath the head so the elbows are pointing outwards.

Movement Execution: This exercise is similar to the one before except that here the legs are not moved up off the ground but the upper body is. The points of the feet are pressed "into" the ground to build up tension in the stretched-out legs, the buttocks and the lower leg. Now lift the upper body up of the ground. Hold this position. The tension in the buttocks and the BS and IC muscles will increase. In order to get an even better training result you tighten the muscles that are being used even more, then loosen up and return to the starting position.

Caution: Once again the same precautions as in the exercises described before are valid. The upper body should not be lifted up too high to avoid too much pressure on the lower back. When moving the upper body upwards, the head should not be pulled back into the neck, it is better to place the chin onto the chest, kind of making a double chin when doing so.

Variation: Here also different positions of the leg are possible. The ankle and the knee can be pulled together or the feet can be spread apart even more. This position once again enables tightening the inside of the upper legs to the maximum. The hands and arms can take up different starting positions. To make it easier, you put them behind the back. *(picture 22a)* or – to work the muscles of the lower back and the buttocks even more – you move the arms in front of the body, either by making a U *(picture 22b)* or by stretching both arms to the side and forwards *(picture 22c)*.

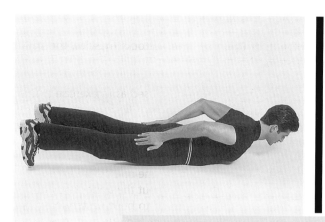

Picture 22a

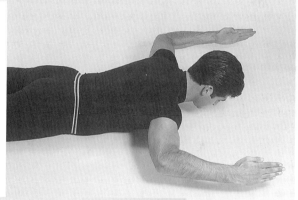

Picture 22b

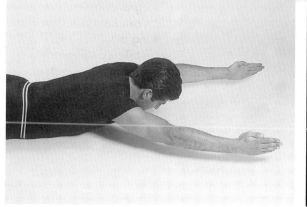

Picture 22c

12. Leg Lift While Sitting on Hands and Knees

Purpose: This exercise puts a strain on the muscles of the buttocks, the pelvic diaphragm, BS and IC muscles.

Starting position: Kneel down on the ground and support your upper body (which is bent forward) with the underarms. Put your weight on the upper thighs, i.e. the right one. Now lift the left knee just a little bit off the ground. The left lower thigh is bent in a right angle to the upper thigh. The foot is flexed, the back straight and the neck is an extension of the spine *(picture 23)*.

Movement Execution: By using the muscles in the buttocks the left leg, leaving it in a right angle, is moved upwards. As soon as the upper thigh is in a horizontal position *(picture 24)* the movement is stopped. Flex all the muscles that need to be trained again and then move the leg back into the starting position. First train one side a couple of times and then the other. You should do the same number of repetitions for each leg.

Caution: If the leg is moved up more than the horizontal position, a hollow back is formed. Please try to avoid this at any case. Hold the pelvis calmly in one position. Do not turn sideways. Furthermore, you should not let the trunk make an evasive movement.

Variation: Numerous variations are possible for this exercise. When in the final position you can make little movements with the bent leg. This increases the tension. If you want to increase the pressure, you can stretch out the leg that you will lift up *(picture 25)* and you can make the above mentioned variation with a stretched out leg as well.

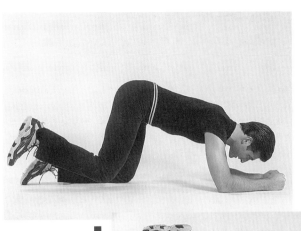

Picture 23

Picture 24

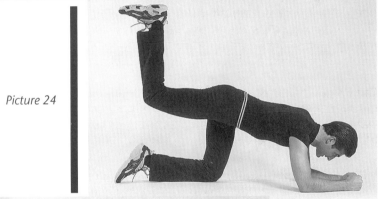

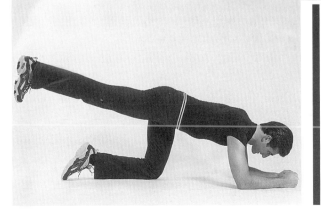

Picture 25

13. Leg Lift While Lying on the Side

Purpose: This excellent exercise strengthens the inner upper thighs, the BS and the IC muscles.

Starting Position: Lie down on the ground sideways and put your head on the lower bent arm. Stretch out the lower leg and pull the foot upward towards the body. Now the upper leg will be bent by 90° and put forward over the lower leg *(picture 26)*. You use the upper hand to prop yourself up front. This way the body is in a stable position.

Movement Execution: Lift the upper stretched leg up from the ground as far as possible by flexing the muscles of the inner upper thigh *(picture 27)* without moving the upper body. In the final position, you increase the tension for a short time and then slowly move the leg back to the starting position. Do not prop your foot on the ground for support or the tension will be lost.

Caution: The foot and the pelvis have to be held vertical to the ground and moved that way as well. Do not support your head with your hand, this could lead to a bending of the spine. It is better to support your upper body with the upper arm up front to stabilise the body posture during the movement.

Variation: Here are also two variations for the stretched out leg. You can either point the foot all the way (pointing) or strongly pull it towards the body (flexing). The upper leg can be placed behind the lower one so the upper foot will come down behind the lower knee. A further variation is to place the back foot in front of the knee of the lower leg.

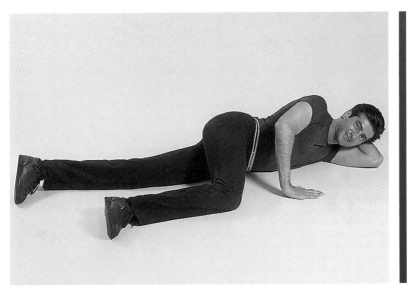

Picture 26

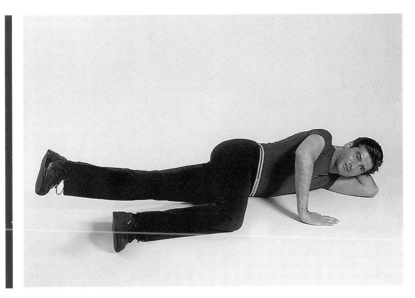

Picture 27

14. Lifting the Leg from a Lateral Position, the Upper Leg Is Bent

Purpose: This exercise also strengthens the inner upper legs, the BS and the IC muscles.

In addition to that, the abductor muscles of the opposite upper thigh are flexed all the time and trained through this.

Starting Position: Take up the same position as in the exercise before. This time both legs are bent 90° and the upper leg will be held up in the air during the whole exercise *(picture 28)*.

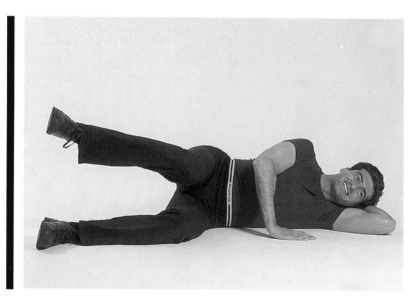

Picture 28

Movement Execution: By flexing the abductors, lift the lower leg off the ground until it touches the upper one *(picture 29)*. Hold this tension and then return to the starting position. Try not to put the lower foot onto the ground.

Caution: The same precaution measures are valid here as in the exercise before.

Variation: Here we also have two variations of how to hold the foot, as described before. A further variation is to stretch both legs *(picture 29a)*.

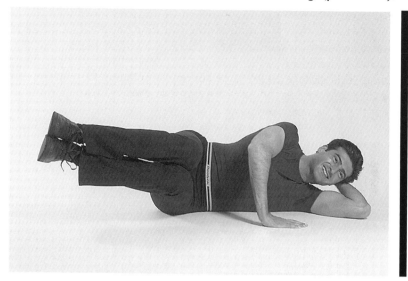

Picture 29

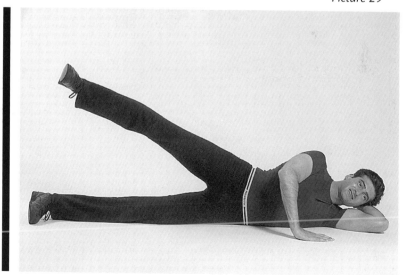

Picture 29a

15. Diagonal Level

Purpose: Maximum stimulation of the muscles of the buttocks, the lower back muscles, the pelvic diaphragm, BS and IC muscles.

Starting Position: Sit down on the ground with your legs stretched out. The hands are propped onto the ground for support, the palms are down, a little more than shoulder-width behind the body. The fingers are pointing in the direction of the buttocks *(picture 30)*.

Movement Execution: Now you move the buttocks as far as possible off the ground so the legs will form one straight line with the upper body *(picture 31)*. The cervical spine is an extension of the whole spine.

Caution: This is a difficult, very intensive exercise!

Variation: To increase the result of this exercise, you can additionally pick up one leg off the ground *(picture 32)*.

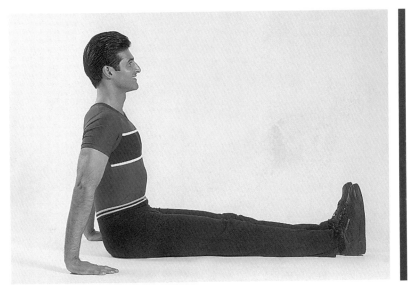

Picture 30

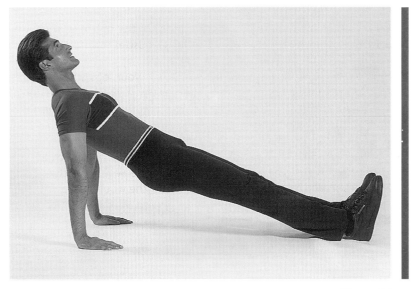

Picture 31

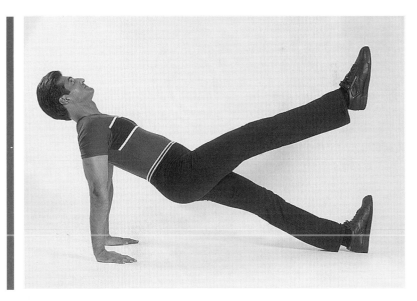

Picture 32

The opponent muscles (antagonists) of those being trained also have to be included in the programme to avoid an imbalance of the muscle system. The exercises before have trained the pelvic region as well as the middle part of the back of the body. Now we want to pay attention to the front middle part of the body.

16. Crunches

Purpose: Muscles of the stomach, especially the upper ones.

Starting Position: Lie down with your back on the floor, spread your legs apart about the width of the pelvis. The points of the feet are pointing upwards. The bend of the knee should be no more than 90°. The hands are crossed behind the head. The elbows are pointing outwards. The chin is bend into a double chin (towards the cervical spine) *(picture 33)*.

Movement Execution: Move the upper body vertebra per vertebra off the ground using the muscles of the stomach. The movement starts with the head and then continues into the upper part of the upper body. The lower back stays on the ground during the whole movement. You remain in the final position *(picture 34)* for a short time and then slowly return to the starting position. If you do not move the upper body back down all the way at the end, a tension remains in the stomach muscles.

Caution: During this exercise it is important that the lumbar spine stays fixed to the ground. Do not use too much swing in this exercise. The head should be an extension of the rest of the spine. This is easier to do if your eyes can focus on one point on the ceiling.

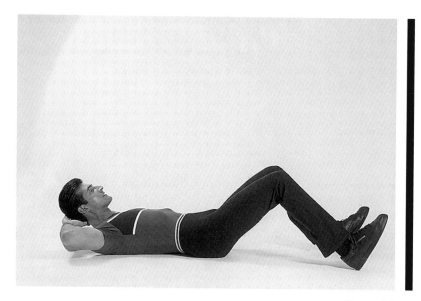

Picture 33

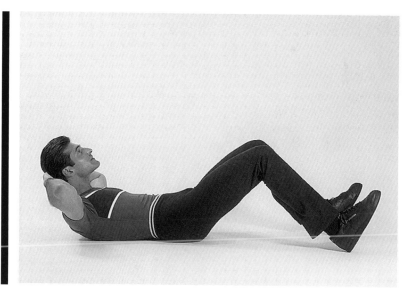

Picture 34

Variation: For some this exercise will be quite difficult at first. Therefore it will be easier to prop a pillow behind your back. The hands behind the head take the strain off the neck muscles. Countless variations for the arms can be used during this exercise. It might be a little easier at the beginning to cross the arms in front of the chest *(picture 34a)* or to stretch and point the arms forward, to the side of the body *(picture 34a1)*.

It will become more difficult when you stretch one arm out and up *(picture 34b)*. The difficulty of this exercise is increased even more if you stretch out both arms upwards. You can also put both arms stretched out behind the head *(picture 34c)* and rest the head on the upper arms.

It is a little bit easier to just hold one arm stretched out behind the head *(picture 34d)*. The feet also can take up different positions. You can simply put the soles of the feet all the way onto the floor *(picture 34e)*.
    A further variation is to bend the legs less *(picture 34e1)*. Always keep them bent a little bit at least. It will be a bit more difficult when you lift the legs that are in a right angle *(picture 34f)*.

You can cross the ankles of the feet or leave them standing parallel to each other. To support the position of the leg here you can place your lower legs onto a chair. The most difficult variation is to stretch the legs almost all the way into the air, while doing so taking one of the positions for the feet as described before.

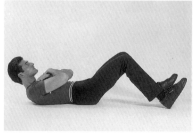

Picture 34a

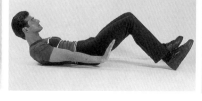

Picture 34a1

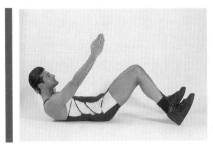

Picture 34b

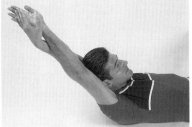

Picture 34c

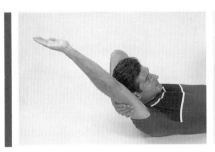

Picture 34d

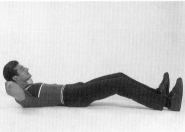

Picture 34e

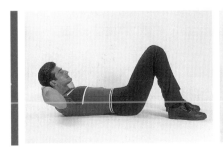

Picture 34e1

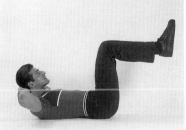

Picture 34f

17. Reverse Crunches

Purpose: Muscles of the stomach, especially the lower ones.

Starting Position: Lie down with your back on the floor, both legs stretched in the air and straightened out almost all the way. Put your arms beside the body *(picture 35)*.

Movement Execution: Slowly move the pelvis off the ground using the help of the lower stomach muscles by pushing the feet up towards the sky or the ceiling. The spine keeps ground contact during the whole movement. Stay in the final position *(picture 36)* and then slowly return to the starting position. The upper body and the arms are not moving.

Caution: During this movement the legs are not to be bent or stretched but the pelvis is supposed to be lifted off the ground. Do not swing. To avoid making a hollow back, you can put your chin on your chest and also actively press the spine onto the ground.

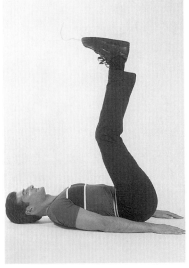
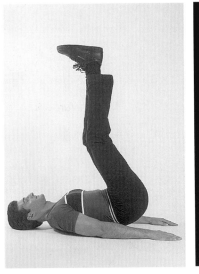

Picture 35   Picture 36

Variation: In order to execute this very difficult exercise more easily, you can bend the legs in the hips and in the knees 90° *(picture 36a)*. In both variations, with stretched or bent knees, you can either hold the feet parallel to each other or cross them. The position of the arms and hands also can be changed. You can hold the hands, just like in the exercise before, behind the head. If this exercise is still difficult even though you use the easier variations, you can use a little trick:

When lying on the back with bent knees, simply put your feet on a chair or bench for support *(picture 37)*. Now the pelvis is lifted *(picture 37a)*. Does this work better? When doing this, the lower back is picked up a little as well so please be careful. And keep remembering: Even one try is training already! Do not give up, soon you will be able to at least do the exercises using the easier variation. And keep in mind that often our stomach muscles are the least developed muscles in our body.

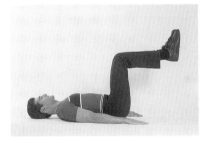

Picture 36a

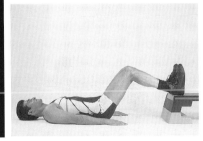

Picture 37

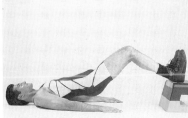

Pictures 37a

18. Jack-knife (Pelvic Lift With Crunch)

Purpose: Training all of the stomach muscles.

Starting Position: For this exercise you also have to lie down with the back on the floor. The knees are bent into a right angle and held in front of the body. The hands are crossed behind the head. The elbows are pointed outwards just like they were in the first exercise for the stomach muscles and the chin is also pulled towards the breastbone *(picture 38)*.

Movement Execution: Lift the upper body, just as in doing crunches, off the ground. At the same time move your pelvis with bent knees, as if doing reverse crunches upward *(picture 39)*. Pay attention to the spine, the lower part should not leave the ground too much. When in the final position, flex all the muscles that are being trained again and then slowly return to the starting position.

Caution: The same precautions are valid here as in exercises 16 and 17.

Variation: All variations that are described before can be combined with each other. Whether you stretch the legs when doing so or change the position of the arms is of no importance at all. Find the right combination for you to effectively use this exercise! You should keep this in mind for all exercises.

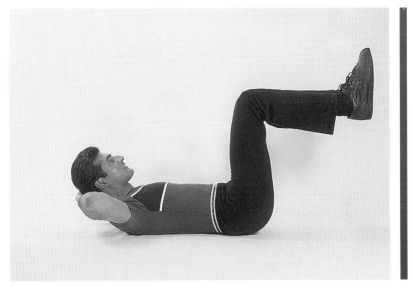

Picture 38

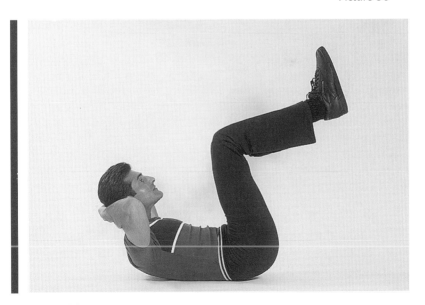

Picture 39

19. Roll Up to the Side

Purpose: The stomach muscles on the side also have to be included to complete the training of the middle part of the body.

Starting Position: You are lying on your back. One leg is positioned across the other, its foot rests on the knee of the other leg. Cross your hands behind the head. The elbows and the chin are taking up the same position as they did in the first exercise *(picture 40)*.

Movement Execution: Turn the upper body and the elbows with the help of the diagonal muscles of the stomach towards the opposite knee. The movement begins with the head and then continues with the upper part of the upper body. The lower part of the back remains on the floor during the whole movement. Remain in the final position for just a short time *(picture 41)* and then slowly return to the starting position. When you have done training one side you switch legs and now turn the upper body towards the other knee.

Caution: The same precautions as for the other stomach muscle exercises are valid.

Variation: The position of the arms can be changed in this exercise, too. Stretch both arms out in front of the body *(picture 41a)*. When moving upward, move one hand through the hole that is created by the angled leg. You can also stretch out one arm and let the other rest behind the neck. Countless arm variations can be used here as well. Let your fantasy run free. But continue to pay attention to the basic movement to be able to do a successful training of the stomach. It is also possible to put both heels onto the ground, then you can take turns turning right and left and by doing so train with each repetition different diagonal stomach muscles.

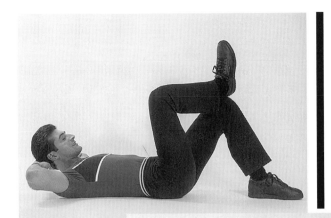

Picture 40

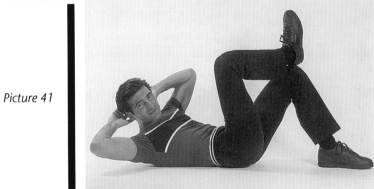

Picture 41

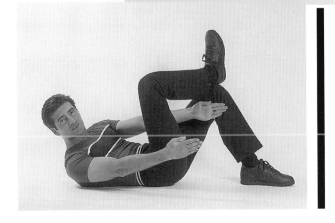

Picture 41a

6.2 Muscle Exercises with Devices

All exercises described above can also be performed against resistance *(picture 41b)*. In the following, we explain about exercises with new variations and new strains. Purpose of the exercises, the starting position, the movement execution, the special instructions, the described variations for the individual exercises, all stays unchanged.

As devices to increase the demand for the muscles that will get trained you can use elastic bands, for example. They are offered in sport stores in different forces of resistance (marked by different colours). You can also get an increase of resistance by using more bands at once.

Different kinds of weights, for example foot cuffs filled with sand, iron shoes, and disc barbells are suitable to be used as auxiliary material. When using these, the resistance can be increased and adjusted well by using heavier weights or multiple foot weights at once.

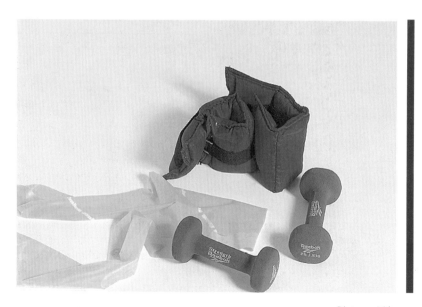

Picture 41b

A. Pelvic Swing

Compare with exercise (1).
When doing this exercise you can place the band across the hip *(picture 42)*. The hands are stretched out and around the band. When swinging the pelvis forwards, the band tightens. To increase the resistance in the end position even more, you can pull your arms backward more. This movement tightens the band even more and the pelvic diaphragm is forced to tighten even more.

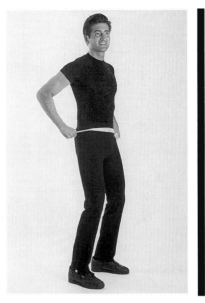

Picture 42

B. Bending the Knee With Pelvic Swing

Compare with exercise (2).
Use the band as described under G.

C. Little Pelvic Lift

Compare with exercise (3).
The starting position is changed in as much as the hands are now holding a band that is led across the hip *(picture 43)*.
When lifting the pelvis, the band tightens. You can also place a disc barbell on the pelvis. When doing this, you must bend the arms that are holding contact to the ground, starting from the elbow to use your hands to avoid the weight from sliding around.

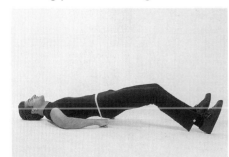

Picture 43

97

D. Little Pelvic Lift With Leg Lift

Compare exercise (4).
For this exercise you can also use a band or a disc barbell to increase the resistance. Furthermore, you can use sand weights for the foot or fasten iron shoes. This increases the strain more.

E. Pelvic Lift

Compare exercise (5).
Please use the disc barbell or the band as described in exercise A *(picture 44)*. When doing the exercise this way, the main difference is that the radius of movement is greater here than in A.

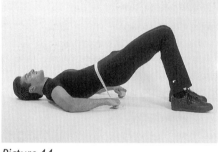

Picture 44

F. Pelvic Lift With Foot Lift

Compare exercise (6).
Use the disc barbell or the band as in the exercise before. In addition to that you can also use the iron shoes or the foot weights to increase the movement resistance *(picture 45)*.

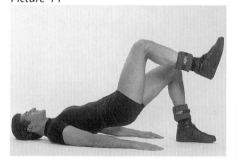

Picture 45

G. Pelvic Lift With Leg Extension

Compare exercise (7)
All is the same as under D *(picture 46)*

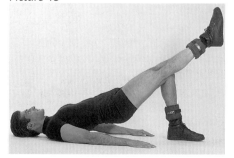

Picture 46

H. Pelvic Lift With Extended Leg

Compare exercise (8).
All remains the same as in exercise D *(picture 47)*.

I. Lifting the Leg from a Prone Position (Boat)

Compare exercise (9)
For this exercise you can use the iron shoes (very difficult!) or the sand filled foot cuffs *(picture 48)*.

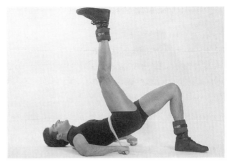

Picture 47

J. Scissors With the Leg Made from a Prone Position

Compare exercise (10).
Please use the resistance as described under I to intensify this exercise.

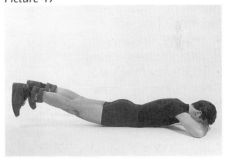

Picture 48

K. Lifting the Trunk from a Prone Position (Cobra)

Compare with exercise (11).
Now you can attach the sand weights around your hands and hold dumbbells in your hand *(picture 49)* or hold a disc barbell behind your head.

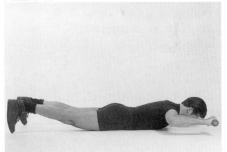

Picture 49

When using a disc barbell, you should always hold them with your hand, in this case the different arm variations cannot be used. When using sand weights or smaller hand dumbbells, however, you can do all arm variations as described under No. 11.

L. Leg Lift While on Hands and Knees

Compare to exercise (12)
An increase of resistance can be accomplished when using weights for the foot *(picture 50)* or iron shoes.

A variation that is a little bit more difficult is the use of the band. You should loop it around the sole of the foot *(picture 50a)*. The other end will be fixed by the knee or held with the hands.
     When moving upward, the band is being tightened.

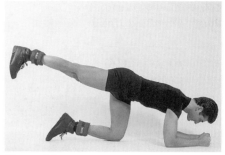

Picture 50

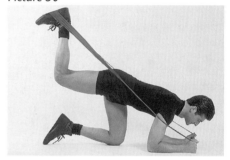

Picture 50a

M. Leg Lift from a Lateral Position

Compare to exercise (13)
For this exercise foot weights *(picture 51)* or iron shoes can also be recommended. The band can also be used to increase resistance.

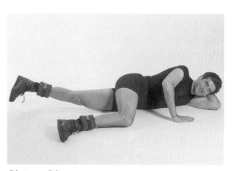

Picture 51

The loop is put around the sole of the foot, the free end attached to the other foot. You can also use the arm that originally was placed underneath the head and move it downwards and hold the band with it.

N. Left Lift from a Lateral Position With Bent Upper Leg

Compare to exercise (14)
For the exercise the upper leg that is being moved upwards should have a foot cuff or an iron shoe attached to it at any rate. In addition to this, the upper leg that is only held can get an additional load with the help of a foot cuff or an iron shoe *(picture 52)*.

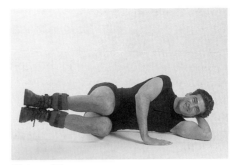

Picture 52

O. Diagonal Gradient

Compare exercise (15).
Lead the band that is stretched diagonally across the pelvis. Both hands hold the ends of the band. The upward movement of the pelvis tightens the band. Resistance is increased by this *(picture 53)*.

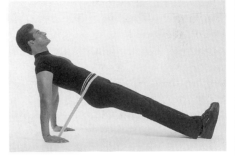

Picture 53

P. Crunches

Compare to exercise (16).
If you fold your hands behind your head during this exercise you can hold a

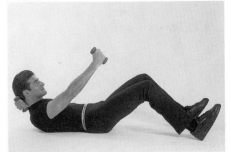

Picture 54

disc barbell there, too. An easier variation is to hold the weight with folded hands above the chest. If you prefer other arm variations as described under No. 16 you should put on weight cuffs around your wrist or use smaller dumbbells *(picture 54)*.

Q. Reverse Crunches

Compare to exercise (17)

During exercises where you hold your legs in the air (almost stretched out all the way or bent a little) you can use foot weights or iron shoes. Because of the additional load on the feet you have to be careful not to make a hollow back.

Instead of the loads on the foot you can simply use the band again. Put the band once around the feet when they are almost stretched out all the way and hold it with your hands that lie parallel to the body on the ground *(picture 55)*. Since the legs are bent about 90° during this exercise, there are two possibilities how to hold the band: You can put it around your knuckle or you use the easier variation and place the band just below your knee.

If you should do this exercise with your hands on a chair, you can either put the band over the pelvis or place disc barbells on it. When using disc barbells you have to bend the arm again to hold the weight during the movements.

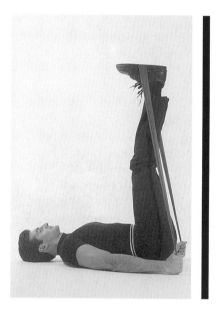

R. Jack-knife (Pelvic Lift With Crunch)

Picture 55

Compare to exercise (18)

The feet can be burdened with weight cuffs or iron shoes. Additionally a disc barbell can be held behind the head or the arms can bear an extra load with weight cuffs as described under P. You can also use the version in which only the arms carry an extra weight. There are no limits set for the possibilities to combine.

S. Roll-up Sideways

Compare to exercise (19).
You can use the load variations as described under P. Different variations for the arms are possible here as well *(picture 56)*.

Coming up, the exercises to train steadiness are described. For these, different machines or a long dumbbell is needed.

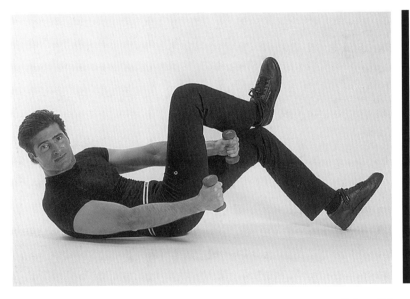

Picture 56

7. Squats

Purpose: The muscles of the buttocks, the pelvic diaphragm, the BS and IC muscles as well as all of the muscles of the upper thigh are being trained here.

Starting Position: Put the long dumbbell behind your neck so it lies on your shoulders. The legs are bent just a little bit. You are standing with your legs about hip-width apart. The feet are bent slightly outward. Keep your eyes focused on one point on the wall at the height of your eyes in order to hold your back straight *(picture 57)*.

Movement Execution: Now start bending your legs until you are in a squatting position *(picture 58)*. Starting from this low position, push yourself back upward in one controlled flowing movement until you are back in the starting position. Pay attention not to lock up your knees in this position. Now move your pelvis forward just like in exercise (1) and flex all muscles that need to be trained.

Caution: People who are not used to working with free dumbbells should first learn how to handle them before using heavy weights. Hold the upper body straight during the whole movement. Try not to bend it forwards because this would put a strong pressure onto the lower part of the spine. If you train together with a partner, he can control your movements. Or you can exercise in front of a mirror to keep an eye on your body posture.

Just like with the leg press, during this exercise you should also never stretch out your legs all the way at the end of the movement. Concentrate on using a slow motion during the exercise, do not use too much swing.

Movement Variations: There are numerous possibilities for training variations. If the ankles of your foot are not flexible enough to leave the soles flat on the ground during the movement execution, you can put a small, solid support (wooden wedge) underneath your heel. You can also change the distance of the feet. The farther they are apart, the more strain is put onto the inner muscles of the upper thigh and the bigger the tension on the BS and IC muscles gets. The movement radius can also be decreased if you just make half or a quarter of a squat instead of a whole one *(picture 59)*. As a rule, the less you bend your knees, the heavier your

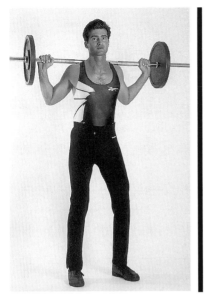

Picture 57

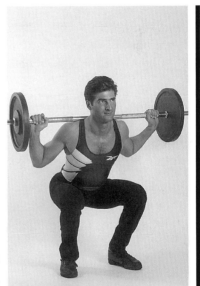

Picture 58

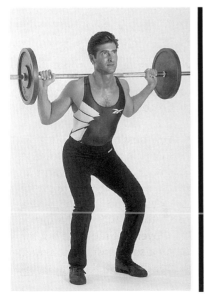

Picture 59

weights can be. The tension in the muscles that need to be trained increases by the movement to lift the pelvis. A squat using the full radius of movement builds up high tension in the muscles, especially when you bring up the weight from a squatting position. Please only practise this exercise with somebody to control it.

A quite difficult variation is to do the squat all the way but only come back up $3/4$ of the way. At the highest point the knee then is still bent quite a bit. Now make the movement to lift the pelvis. This is quite difficult! You muscles must work as hard as they can.

You choose an even more demanding variation if the pelvic lift is made in the starting position already. Now slowly go down to a squat with the pelvic lift forward. You will not be able to go down quite as much as you would without the pelvic lift forward. Do you feel just how hard the pelvic diaphragm is working?

You can also do squats on the machine. The machine makes sure you stick to vertical movements. This prevents making evasive movements. The back is held straight. But the intensity of this training is also lowered when using this variation. For starters it is especially suitable to learn the movement execution.

Finally a little tip:
Use a padding to reduce the pressure on your shoulders! It is much more pleasant to train this way! But be careful that the dumbbell will not roll backwards.

U. Leg Press

Purpose: The same muscles are being activated here as with the squat except that the lower back and the upper torso do not have to use as much energy to stabilise the dumbbell. This way it is easier to concentrate on the muscles that need to be exercised.

Starting Position: Adjust the backrest and the seat so when the feet go in their place the knees are bent. The points of the feet are pointing outward. The weight should be brought down as much as possible by bending the knees as much as possible. The knees are bending in the direction that the feet are pointing towards (*picture 60*).

Movement Execution: Stretch out your legs until the knees are straightened out almost all the way *(picture 61)*. From this position you lift your pelvis forward just like when doing the squat that was explained before and you tighten the pelvic diaphragm. Then you bend your legs again and get back to the starting position.

Caution: Do not get in the habit of pressing your hands onto the kneecaps or upper thighs when pressing the weight up.

Movement variations: Depending on the way the bench press is built, it is possible to change the distance of the foot. Here the same rules are valid as when doing squats. The further the feet are apart, the more tension is built up in the adductors. When using the leg press you can keep the pelvis lifted during the whole movement to get the maximum stimulation for the pelvic diaphragm. This is a difficult exercise!

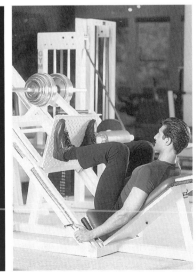
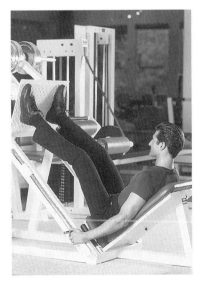

Picture 60   Picture 61

V. Cable Pull to the Inside/Adductor Machine

Purpose: Adductors, pelvic diaphragm, BS and IC muscles.

Starting Position: Go to the cable pull machine.
Put on the padded foot loop. Stand sideways, a couple of centimetres away from the weights of the machine and hold onto the handgrip of the machine (on the post). The leg that is closer to the machine is turned outwards about 45° *(picture 62)*. The point of the foot points downwards. You can feel a certain tension in this leg. Now lift your pelvis up forwards.

Movement Execution: Now the foot of the stretched out leg is being moved in front of the supporting leg towards the middle of the body *(picture 63)* and a little bit beyond that. Hold this position for a short time and then increase the lifting movement of the pelvis forward. Increase the tension and now move the stretched out leg back to the starting position.

Caution: Try to avoid evasive movements of the hip and the upper torso. The upper torso should remain upright during the whole movement.

Movement Variations: Many studios have adductor machines. By moving the upper thighs together at the same time they increase the tension in the pelvic diaphragm, especially at the end of the movement.

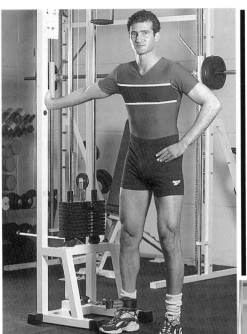

Picture 62

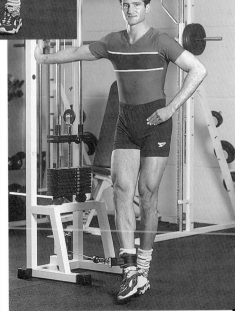

Picture 63

7 Exercises and Training Methods to Increase the Blood Flow (Circulation) and Oxygen Support in the Penis

During all strength and endurance training exercises you should avoid using machines that causes perineal pressure (onto the region between the testicle and the anus). This would cause a reduced blood supply to the penis.

7.1 Strength Exercises

You should use weights using 75-85% of the maximum strength to keep up the optimum increase of circulation going during the breaks and in between the sets as well.

Once again we must emphasise that you should warm up well before using heavy weights. It is also very important to take breaks of about 3 minutes and 30 seconds length between the individual sets not to disturb the increased circulation that has been caused by the exercise.

When exercising the circulation and oxygen support improvement you should make sure that your movements are speedy all the time, this is quite a difference to the muscle training as described before which has the primary goal to strengthen the pelvic diaphragm, and the IC and BS muscles. But the exercises should not be performed too fast and uncontrolled.

I. Leg Press

Main Load: This movement can be made on totally different leg presses. Roughly differentiated there are three kinds of machines:

On the first one you lie down on your back and push the weights vertically up with your feet.

Then there is the variation where you push the weights forward parallel to the ground from a sitting position. And there is another machine from which the weight is pushed diagonally upwards on a track that is angled about 45°.

Regardless of the kind of the machine, the result always is a strong increase of the blood circulation in the penis. In the breaks the rates of blood flowing through it are about the amount as during an erection.

In addition the muscles of mainly the front upper thighs and secondarily the ischiocrural muscles and those of the buttocks are being exercised.

Starting Position: The feet are put against the foot holders of the machine, the knees are bent. The points of the feet are pointing outward. The weight should be moved down as much as possible. The knees are bent in the direction that the toes are pointing.

Movement Execution: Stretch out your legs, straightening the knees almost all the way. Then bend the legs again to get back to the starting position.

Caution: Never stretch out the legs all the way at the end of the movement. The same precaution measures as described in exercise (V) are valid.

Movement Variation: Depending on the kind of leg press, you can change the distance of the feet. You can bring the ankles of the feet and the knees together; this increases the strain on the muscles of the buttocks.

When moving the legs and feet further apart, the activity in the inner upper thigh muscles is increased.

II. Squat

Main Strain: This is the best exercise to increase the blood circulation in the penis. If it is performed right, it is very strenuous and a lot of strength is needed for it. The front upper thighs, the ischiocrural muscles, the muscles of the buttocks, back extensors and stomach muscles are being exercised.

Starting Position: Put the barbell stick onto the knee-bend rack and attach the wanted weights. Now move underneath the long dumbbell that is still on the rack so the bar lies behind your neck on the shoulders. Now you grab the bar and lift it from its rack. The feet are slightly turned outward.

Movement Execution: Now bend your legs until you are in a squatting position. Some people will advise you not to squat down this deep. But if you do not have any problems before and do this exercise purposely without swing and without rocking up and down when squatting, there are no reservations against it. Starting from the deepest point you go back into the starting position in a controlled and flowing movement.

Caution: Please read the precautionary measures as described under exercise (T.).
Just like with the leg press you should not straighten out your legs all the way at the end of the movement here, either.

Movement Variation: You can do all variations as described in exercise T. here as well. But notice that a decrease of the movement radius will also cause a decrease of the penile circulation in the breaks.

You can also do the squat holding the weight on your chest *(picture 64)*. Naturally, when doing this, you cannot handle the same heavy weights as when the weight is behind the neck. The muscles of the front upper thighs are also used more during this exercise. When picking up the dumbbell you either grab it with the hands at shoulder's width or with the arms crossed in front of the chest, the elbows must be held up *(picture 65)*.

You can also do the squats on the machine. Details about this can be read under T. A rather seldom variation is a squat where mainly the lower upper thigh muscles are being worked on. The circulation of the penis is not as pronounced during this exercise as when during the original squat.

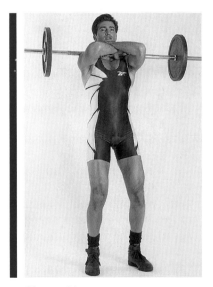

Picture 64

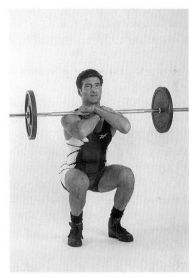

Picture 65

III. Leg Extension

Main Strain: The demand lies almost exclusively isolated on the muscles of the front upper thigh. The improvement of the blood circulation of the penis is not as high during this exercise as it is when doing the leg press or the squat.

Starting Position: Sit down on the seat of the leg extension machine so the popliteal cavity is at the edge of the seat. Put the span of your feet underneath the rolls. The hands hold onto the edges of the side of the seat *(picture 66)*.

Movement Execution: Stretch out your legs until the knees are straightened out *(picture 67)*. Remain in this final position for a short time and then intensively tighten the upper thighs. Then return to the starting position.

Caution: After stretching do not swing back and forth in the final position, this can cause damage to the knee-joint.

Movement Variation: The feet can point inward or outward. Depending on the way the toes are pointing, the tension in the muscles of the front upper thighs changes. A further variation is to pull the feet together or to move the toes away as much as possible from the body.

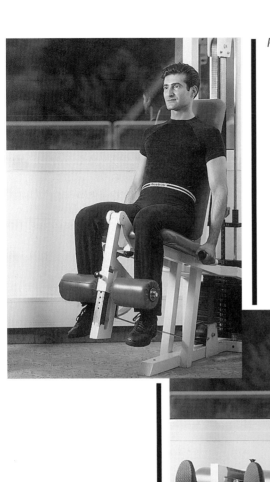

Picture 66

Picture 67

IV. Leg Curls

Main Strain: The emphasis of this exercise is training the back of the upper thighs. The improvement of blood circulation in the penis is about the same as when doing leg stretches.

Starting Position: Lie down flat on your stomach on the leg curl machine and put your heels under the lever mechanism. The legs are stretched. The hands hold onto the side edges of the padding or the hand grips *(picture 68)*.

Movement Execution: Bend your legs as much as possible without lifting the pelvis off the bench *(picture 69)*. After holding it in the final position for a short moment, bring the weight back into the starting position.

Caution: Always keep contact with the bench, do not pick up your buttocks from the bench when pulling the weight up.

Movement Variation: During this exercise you can also lift the point of the feet, stretch them or turn them to the inside or outside. Some studios have a special leg curl machine on which the exercise can only be done standing using one leg at a time.

This might make a lot of sense when trying to build up isolated muscles, but you are working on increasing the blood circulation in the penis. So, please refrain from this variation. There are also leg curl machines you can train on in a sitting position *(picture 70)*. This is a good alternative to avoid the possible danger of damaging your back when lying down *(picture 71)*.

Some fitness trainers will recommend that you put your elbows on the padding for support on the horizontal leg curl machines so the lower part of the body can stay tight on the bench. I do not recommend this variation because a high strain is caused on the lumbar spine when bending the lower leg. This is at most an exercise for well-trained people.

Picture 68

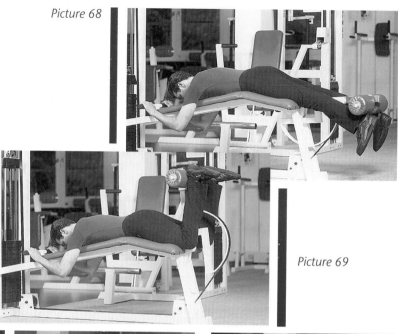

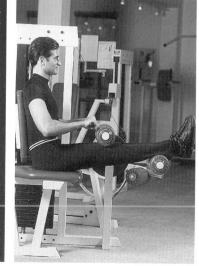

Picture 69

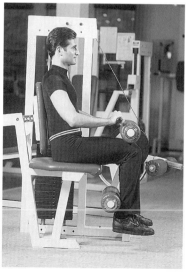

Picture 70

Picture 71

V. Adductor Machine

Main Strain: A very strong strain is put onto the adductors here. The circulation of the penis is about the same as it is during the two exercises described before.

Starting Position: Sit down on the seat of the machine and move your legs outwards. You feel a certain tension in the adductors *(picture 72)*.

Movement Execution: Now you move the almost stretched out legs back together *(picture 73)*. Remain still for a short time and then bring the legs back to the starting position.

Caution: Do not over-stretch the adductors when moving the legs apart.

Movement Variation: You can also train on a machine as described under V (chapter 6.2). But since it is only possible to train one leg at a time, overall the blood circulation and the oxygen supply of the penis is lower here than it is on the adductor machine.

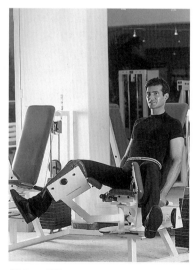

Picture 72

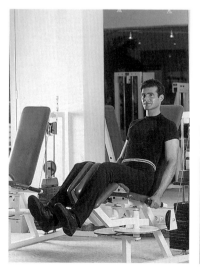

Picture 73

7.2 Endurance Training Using the Interval Principle

7.2.1 General Information

What Is Endurance?
Endurance in sports is defined as the ability to be resistant against getting tired when under a long lasting strain, and a fast recovery afterwards.

Depending on the kind of energy production, we distinguish between aerobic and anaerobic. What does this mean? Aerobic means that there is a sufficient amount of oxygen during energy production. This means that the muscles that are being worked on need little oxygen for the energy production so the oxygen being transported via bloodstream is sufficient. Anaerobic, on the other hand, means that the energy production is caused without oxygen meaning that the transported oxygen is not enough for the energy production, so additional metabolism processes are needed for the energy production without using extra oxygen. This is the so-called oxygen debt.

Measuring the Intensity
Before starting the training, some pre-conditions have to be cleared up or explained. You already know that you have to be warmed-up first. During the warm-up the body should have a strain of no more than 50-60% of its heart capacity. But how do you know that your are really moving within this frame? Sometimes the body plays a joke on you and lets you feel wrong about it. Sometimes you do not even notice if you overstrain yourself. Therefore it is recommendable not only to pay attention to the feeling you get but to also use an objective parameter like the heart rate. So, please check your heart rate! How else would you know that you are at 50-70% of your maximum endurance capacity, for example?

The more intensive you put a strain on the muscles, the higher the demand for oxygen will be. Therefore you will need values for the oxygen demand in order to find out the intensity you are training in right now. But it would not be very practical at all to check the oxygen demand during training. Large medical apparatus would have to be used for this. So, which ways are available to you at all times? The heart rate! And how is the heart rate connected to the oxygen intake?

An important point of the aerobic performance capacity is the maximum oxygen intake. This depends especially on the cardiac output, the capacity of the blood to transport oxygen and the capacity of the working muscles to make use of the oxygen. Training endurance often is measured in "percent of the maximum oxygen intake". Because this indirectly depends on the heart rate, the frequency of the pulse is used as a measurement indicator. This is the most practical way to control the intensity of the training that is available to us.

The proportion between the percentage of the maximum pulse – as a measurement of training intensity – and the percentage of the maximum intake of oxygen is shown in the table below:

% maximum pulse	% maximum oxygen intake
50	28
60	42
70	56
80	70
90	83
100	100

Table 1: Relation between the percentage of the maximum pulse as a training intensity and the percentage of the maximum oxygen intake

How Do I Check My Pulse Rate?

If you do not have a gauge to measure the pulse rate, you have to learn how to check the pulse rate with your fingers. Sometimes, when you are out of breath, it might be difficult to find the pulse and count it.

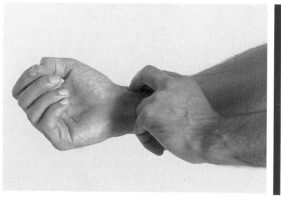

Picture 74

You need a clock showing the seconds. Then there are three good ways to check your pulse on your body.

1. On the forearm (radial pulse): Stretch out your wrist and feel the pulse with the other hand on the side of the thumb between the tendon of the hand and the bone *(picture 74).*
2. On the common carotid artery (carotid pulse): Feel the pulse lateral to the larynx and the edge of the neck muscle.
3. On the temple (temporal pulse): For unpractised people here it is the most difficult place to find the pulse. Put a little bit of pressure onto the temple. If you do not find the pulse right away, simply feel around the temple a little bit.

Once you have found the pulse, look at the clock for 10 seconds and count the pulse beats in this time frame. Multiply them by six and then you get the amount of pulse beats per minute.

How Do I Figure Out My Training Pulse?
There are multiple formulas to determine the training pulse.

For untrained people this is a rough estimate:

Training pulse (in beats/minute) = 180 – age

To make a difference between beginners and people who have been training regularly, you can use a more detailed formula:

Training pulse = 60% of the maximum pulse (lowest values)
Training pulse = 80% of the maximum pulse (highest values)

Those who have just started to work-out should concentrate on the lower values. People who train regularly should concentrate on the higher values. The maximum pulse here is defined as the highest one medically justifiable and it is calculated this way:

Maximum pulse = 220 – age

To explain this calculation a little, we give two examples:

1. Example:
Figuring out the training pulse of a 40-year old, untrained man:

$$(220 - 40) \times 60\% = 108 \text{ beats/minute}$$

2. Example:
Figuring out the training pulse for a 30-year old trained man:

$$(220 - 30) \times 80\% = 152 \text{ beats/minute}$$

According to this for the 40-year old untrained male the pulse beat per minute should not be more than 108 during training, the borderline for a trained 30 year-old male should be at 152 pulse beats per minute.

The best way to get the training pulse is by using the following formula:

$$\text{Training pulse} = (\text{maximum pulse} - \text{resting pulse rate}) \times \text{percentage of training} + \text{resting pulse rate}$$

The resting pulse rate should be measured before getting out of bed in the morning. The maximum pulse is the difference between 220 and the individual age.

For the untrained 40-year old with a resting pulse rate of 64 beats/minute this means:

$$(180 - 64) \times 60\% + 64 = 133 \text{ beats/minute} = \text{the optimal training pulse.}$$

Age	Maximum Pulse	50%	60%	70%
15	205	103	123	143
20	200	100	120	140
25	195	98	117	136
30	190	95	114	133
35	185	93	111	129
40	180	90	108	126
45	175	88	105	122
50	170	85	102	119
55	165	83	99	115
60	160	80	96	112
65	155	78	93	108
70	150	75	90	105
75	145	73	87	101
80	140	70	84	98

Table 2: Maximum pulse depending on the age and the load percentages

Self Assessment of the Load Intensity

The subjective feeling you get for the load intensity that you can handle indeed is a valuable and supplementary aid. But, as mentioned before, it sometimes can be difficult to judge yourself right. If at all, trained people that are already quite experienced with regard to endurance training can judge the physical load relatively well.

With the help of a scale the individual subjective feeling can be assigned to a training strain. It is recommended that you stay in a region between 12 to 16.

Scale	Subjective Feeling
6	
7	very, very easy
8	
9	very easy
10	
11	quite easy
12	
13	a little bit difficult
14	
15	difficult
16	
17	quite difficult
18	
19	very, very difficult
20	

Table 3: Subjective measurement of the intensity of training in accordance with the BORG-scale

A visible sign of a too high intensity is if the colour of the face is dark red. If a white mouth-nose-triangle is also showing, an acute circulatory collapse is about to happen. A decrease of the ability to co-ordinate also is a sign of a too high physical strain. If it is not possible to talk anymore, it is probably due to overstraining, too. Excessive sweating can be a sign of a too high training load for beginners. If a dry cough develops during or after the training this also could be an indication of a too intensive training.

7.2.2 Suitable Types of Sports

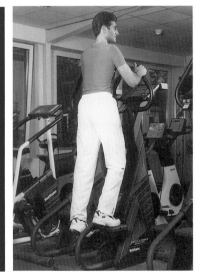

Picture 75

Different types of sports like rowing, running, stair climbing (stepper) *(picture 75)* and bicycling are suitable for interval training. When cycling only the use of a recumbent bicycle shows the effect wished for. When cycling on a normal city bike, on the ergometer and especially on a racing bike with its very hard saddle, the oxygen support of the penis is even more decreased. This is because the point of the saddle squeezes off the blood support to the penis. So, therefore please avoid sitting on a hard saddle!

Out of the four types of endurance sports mentioned above, the interval training on the recumbent bicycle is the most effective one for the penile circulation. The same effect can also be accomplished when intensively climbing stairs or running as interval training. The results that rowing as a sport for the whole body causes are not quite as good. The explanation for this is: when looking at the vascular supply of the penis *(figure 8)*, one sees that all penile vessels start from bigger blood vessels that eventually are responsible for the blood supply of the upper thigh muscles. When intensively training the upper thigh muscles, the distribution of the blood changes. After the end of the training and with it the strain, all vessels are opening up again and the outer genitals get "over-circulated". This effect is only caused when the strain is put purposely on the upper thigh. Rowing, however, puts a strain on the whole body and not exclusively onto the legs. Therefore the increase of the circulation during the rest interval is not quite as extreme as it is when doing sports for the legs only.

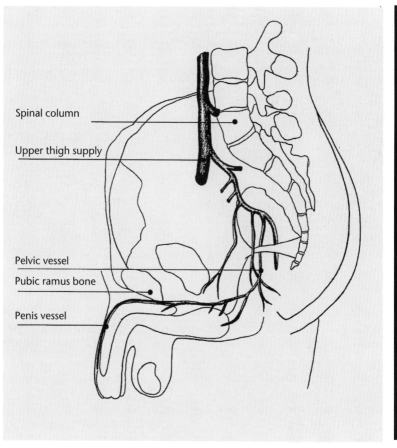

Spinal column

Upper thigh supply

Pelvic vessel

Pubic ramus bone

Penis vessel

Figure 8: Vessel Support of the Penis

In the following paragraphs we want to explain how the blood supply in the penis can be increased with the help of a program that was developed for the stationary training on the recumbent bicycle . Personally, I prefer training on a recumbent bicycle to the stepper or running.

7.3 Interval Training Program

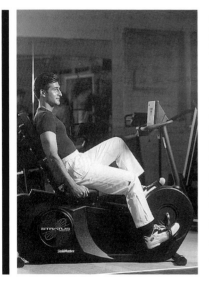

Picture 76

After this excursion into sport physiology we now go back to the training on the recumbent bicycle *(picture 76).*

An important hint beforehand: Beginners that show signs of exhaustion (see chapter 5.4) should stop the training and lightly finish with cycling. For the following interval training a good basic physical condition is needed. The goal of the program is to get a maximum oxygen debt and to get a local overacidification in the muscles of the upper thighs.

After cycling slowly for about 10-15 minutes, and hopefully having warmed up well, you start with the first interval. Start cycling and try to reach 85-90% of your top performance. Try to keep this speed constantly for two minutes. Are you all worn out now? – Then you should cycle slowly again. Continue to cycle for five minutes using 50-60% of your top capacity.

After that you start the hard training again and go to 85-90% of your maximum capacity for two minutes. This is quite strenuous. Now try again to get the heart rate back down to 50-60% of your maximum training intensity for five minutes. You repeat the two minutes exertion with the five minutes breaks a total of three times again. After the last load interval you can leisurely finish cycling so your heart rate slowly goes down towards the resting value. The circulation of the penis after this strenuous interval training is at its maximum. So therefore please do not take a cold shower right away but first relax for a certain amount of time.

An Overview of the Program Is Shown Here:

Time in minutes	Training phase	Load in per cent of the maximum pulse
10 - 15	warm-up	50 - 60
2	strain	85 - 90
5	recovery	50 - 60
2	strain	85 - 90
5	recovery	50 - 60
and so on: a total of five straining phases		
7 - 10	cool-down	

This program puts a great demand on your cardiovascular system. If you are not used to doing endurance sports, you should first build up a certain basic endurance to be able to go through this strenuous interval training. You are probably asking yourself now how you can build up a basic endurance capability? – By first regularly training 30-50 minutes on the recumbent bicycle or by running 7-10 kilometres on a regular basis.

To come back to our program example with the recumbent bicycle: It stands to reason that a basic endurance capacity is necessary for the strenuous interval training in order to quickly recover after the high strain for two minutes, so you can meet the challenge again after five minutes.

If the two minutes are too strenuous and the training volume is too much for you, you can choose any time you like between 30 seconds and two minutes. If you want to, you can also lower the active resting phases to

3:30-5 minutes if the endurance time before is shortened, it all depends on your physical condition. If you do not have a lot of time for the training, you could use the following training:

You begin by warming-up for 10 minutes. Then do 40 seconds strain (power) so you get close to 85-90% of your maximum physical performance. After that do 3:30 minutes calm physical movement, so that you reach about 50-60% of your maximum training heart rate. Then do another 40 seconds long power phase.

The same recovery phase as before is observed now and this interval is repeated once again. After that comes the cool-down phase for a duration of between 5-7 minutes. So you do not need more than 30 minutes to do a little favour to the circulation and oxygen support of your penis.

8 Training for Beginners

In this chapter some programs are suggested to you. Once you have gathered more experience with this training, you can make up your own program.

But first get familiar with the programs recommended. Later you can replace individual exercises by others that you might prefer. The already described repertoire of exercises (chapter 9.1, 9.2 and 10) is large.

Please always pay attention to the following basic rules:

■ The exercises should be put together in a logical order. We cannot emphasise enough that in a complete program the steadiness always has to be exercised first and after that the exercises to increase the circulation of the blood.

■ Do not force anything. If the execution of the exercise does not really work too well, you can simply use an easier variation. And keep the motto that we have repeated here often already, in mind: Giving it a try is training already.

■ Get used to a set program before you change anything. Once you are quite familiar with this program you do not constantly have to think about what exercise comes next and how to execute it. If you are familiar with the program, it is much easier to focus your energy on the muscles that need to be trained, or the circulation.

8.1 General Information

At first please carefully read this book to get familiar with the exercises and the principles of training. So, therefore, please do not storm into the exercise basement or the fitness studio without really comprehending what you want to do. The result would be that you do not accomplish the results wished for and do not reach the goals set.

This would lead you to becoming frustrated, losing interest in training and finally become a bored couch potato again. And this again would not really promote your potency! If you are inattentive or negligent you can

131

hurt yourself. What is needed to get going well from the beginning, I will tell you in the following sentences.

First of all you have to understand the basic terms of training theory.

8.2 Basic Terms

The *exercise* is a movement that you make during training. There is a starting position from which the movement is started and often there is a final position from which you return to the starting position.

The *repetition* is the full movement process of an exercise in its individual execution.

A *set* is the group of repetitions that is made without a break. When training for steadiness, for example, an exercise should be repeated 8-15 times without a break. Usually each movement is performed in a set.

A *rest interval* is the time in between the sets that you give the muscles that are being trained right then to recover. Depending on the training condition, the duration is between one and two minutes. The rest interval should be longer according to your training condition (if you are untrained and the exercise strenuous, the rest intervals should be longer).

The *training program* includes all exercises, repetitions and sets that are made in one training session (workout).

The *contraction* means the flexing of the muscles. If you touch the muscle that is contracted, you feel that it is getting harder. We differentiate between isotonic contractions and isometric ones.

During the isotonic contraction, the muscles that are being trained not only tighten but also change in length during the movement execution. During the isometric contraction, a tension of the muscle is built up, the length and the angle of the muscle hereby do not change.

The *weight* (barbell discs *resistance* or *load*, changeable weights on the machines) that you move is called resistance or load.

The *intensity* describes the extent of effort needed to execute the exercise or the effort during the whole training unit. This means that the intensity is increased when using a heavier weight, a higher contraction or when shortening the rest intervals.

We distinguish between two types of training: I have mentioned the term aerobic and anaerobic before already. Aerobic training is a not too intensive training that uses oxygen to get energy. A purely aerobic training increases the endurance and a basic endurance is needed to successfully accomplish the **VigorRobic®** training program. Anaerobic training is high-intensity training. During this the oxygen demand of the body for the energy production is not fully covered anymore. There are metabolic processes happening in the muscles which set energy free without using up any oxygen. It stands to reason that you cannot keep up an anaerobic endurance for a long time because you soon reach your physical performance limits.

8.3 Training for Steadiness

There are four possibilities to increase the load during the exercises:
  1. You increase the weight or the resistance that you use.
  2. You increase the number of repetitions.
  3. You shorten the breaks in between the individual sets.
  4. You increase the training volume as a whole by doing more sets.

You should do at least 8-15 repetitions of the exercises without any tools. If you do not have any problems in doing more repetitions, you should add an additional weight load or use the elastic bands. This means that first the number of repetitions of an exercise should be increased. Once the highest recommended amount of repetitions is reached, you should increase the resistance. Doing so, the number of repetitions should be reduced again. This resistance then should be used until you reach the recommended upper level of the repetitions again. After that you increase the resistance again and so forth.

In order to train for steadiness, it is recommended to increase the resistance after reaching a certain amount of repetitions to increase the training load. The breaks should not be shortened if this is the training goal.

At the beginning you will only be able to do one set of each exercise. After an acclimatisation phase that should last 3-4 weeks, you can slowly add one set to each exercise. If you can do two sets of all exercises you should keep this training volume for 2-3 weeks and take on another set per exercise. When doing so, please do all sets of one exercise first before switching to the next. Do not execute all exercises after another like when doing circle training and then start a new round. So please do not do one exercise after the other as if you do circular training and then start the second round!

An important training method is the **highest contraction.**
A muscle consists of many small muscle fibers that again consist of individual cells. A certain movement activates the cells or not. An activated cell always gives a maximum performance. But why do we all have different strengths? – The more cells are activated, the more power is set free. Exercising makes more sense the more muscle cells are activated simultaneously during a movement. During the pelvic lift, for example, the pelvic diaphragm is activated most in the final position, in which the buttocks are farthest away from the ground. This highest contraction is most effective if the muscles that are to be trained are additionally flexed in the final position. When training for steadiness you have to keep this principle in mind and definitely apply it to get the optimal results.

8.4 Training for Circulation

When training for circulation with weights the same basic rules as explained above during the training for steadiness apply. Between the sets during the breaks there is a surplus of blood circulation in the penis. Therefore it is important to use resistances of 75–85% of the maximum of weights that can be handled and to observe the breaks of 3:30 minutes. Do not take a shorter break! This would have a negative effect on the penile circulation. If the state of exhaustion is too high you can increase the duration of the break.

The number of repetitions that you can do using 75-85% of the maximum allowable weight is between four and eight. Before working with these heavy weights, you should warm up the body well. At first execute the exercises with lighter weights so you can do 15-20 repetitions. If the muscles and the tendons are warmed up well then, you can start the actual training with the heavier weights.

Increasing the weight, the amount of sets and the volume of the training should be organised according to the above mentioned hints. If eight repetitions can easily be done with a weight, you should increase the next training session so you can only do four or five repetitions with it.

When training according to the interval endurance method it is important that you nearly wear yourself out during the power phase. The active rest intervals between the power phases should last at least 3 minutes and thirty seconds or, depending on the condition, five minutes or even longer. Active rest interval means that, for example, when walking on a stepper the power phase of this movement is continued as calmly as needed to catch your breath again. Once you have recovered and feel fit again, you start the next power phase.

8.5 The Right Body Posture and Movement Execution

You should get used to paying attention to the right body posture and movement execution during all exercises. Try to only move those parts of the body that are mentioned in the individual descriptions of the exercises.

If other parts of the body help out, this is called distortion, an incorrect execution that happens especially to beginners and definitely has to be corrected.

The speed of the exercise execution during strength training depends on whether you want to train for steadiness or for circulation.

When training for steadiness, a slow movement using all of your movement ability enables an optimum stimulation of the muscles. Also using weights and making slow movements (medium acceleration of an inertial mass) hinders the muscles from becoming relieved which would happen due to the impulse rapid movements would cause. Velocity plays an important role during the individual repetitions as well.

The upward movement should last 2-4 seconds, the downward movement 3-5 seconds. The longer the distance, the longer is the movement execution. When squatting to train the steadiness 4 seconds should be used for the upward movement. You should remain at the final position for a short time and then slowly go back to a squat. For the downward movement you should use five seconds.

For the exercise "pelvic lift", shorter distances are covered than when squatting. Therefore you can get from the starting position to the final position in two seconds. There you remain still at first and then lower the pelvis for three seconds.

The slower down movement of the weights and the moving back of the body to the starting position has two advantages: Due to the slow negative phase of the movement, the muscles strongly contract again and because of this, the risk of injuring the muscles, tendons or joints is lowered.

When training to increase the circulation, it is important to do speedy, flowing movements. The exercise execution should be faster than when training the steadiness, but nevertheless controlled. Here bringing the weights down or moving the body back to the starting position should be slower than the upward movement.

8.6 Rest Intervals

When training the steadiness, you should try to keep rest intervals of 60-120 seconds in between the sets. The body stays warm in this time so there is no increased risk of getting injured when starting the next set. The muscles can recover sufficiently during this duration in order to be ready again for the next set.

During the circulation and oxygen training it is important to obey the rest intervals of at least three minutes and thirty seconds between the individual sets because in the rest periods, the wished for higher blood circulation of the outer genitalia is reached.

8.7 Breathing

It is best to exhale during the systolic time interval. In the returning or relaxing phase you inhale again. At the beginning you have to think about how to breathe. But after a couple of training units at least, you will automatically breathe correctly. Keep in mind that during the positive strenuous phase you cannot hold your breath. This means you should try to avoid compressed breathing.

When doing interval training, you have to inhale more air into your lungs because you need much more oxygen here than during the rest interval. You can accomplish this excess demand by inhaling and exhaling more quickly and by taking deeper breaths. You breathe in deeper and faster. During the warm-up, the interval and the cool-down phase you should actively support the respiration process.

When running, climbing stairs (stepper), cycling and rowing, try to breathe in and out deeply and regularly in the rhythm of your leg or rowing movement. Try, for example, to breathe in through your nose for the duration of three steps when running and to exhale through your mouth during the following three steps. You should always inhale through your nose because the air that is breathed in is moistened better this way, warmed up and cleaned. During the intervals, meaning during the power phases, you should use a combination of inhaling through your nose and mouth.

8.8 Frequency of Training

If you want to combine training for steadiness and for blood circulation with an increase of oxygen intake in one training session, training three times a week is sufficient. You should try to rest at least 48 hours between the individual training days to recover well.

You can also split up the training for steadiness as well as the training of the circulation by doing the exercises for steadiness one day and the training for circulation the next. Here you should also train both three times a week. This would mean that you get six training sessions a week, a program that I can recommend only for well-trained people. You should definitely use the only interval day of the week accordingly! Do not continue to train without a break!

8.9 Training Programs

Below I show you what a complete training program for beginners or men who have not been doing any sports in quite a while can look like:

Exercises	Time/Sets	Intensity/Reps.	Recommendations
I Warm-up Recumbent bicycle	10 min	low intensity	50-60% of capacity
II Steadiness			
Pelvic swing	1 Set	10 times	no resistance
Pelvic lift	1 Set	10 times	no resistance
Leg scissors from a prone position	1 Set	12 times	no resistance
Leg Press	1 Set	18 times	50% of max. weight
Adductor machine	1 Set	13 times	60% of max. weight
Reverse crunches	1 Set	15 times	no resistance
Crunches	1 Set	20 times	no resistance

III Circulation			
Recumbent bicycle	2 min	low intensity	50-60% of perf. capacity
Recumbent bicycle	30 sec	high intensity	85-90% of perf. capacity
Recumbent bicycle	3:30 min	low intensity	50% of perf. capacity
Recumbent bicycle	30 sec	high intensity	85-90% of perf. capacity
Recumbent bicycle	3:30 min	low intensity	50% of perf. capacity
Recumbent bicycle	30 sec	high intensity	85-90% of perf. capacity
IV Cool down			
Recumbent bicycle	6 min	low intensity	50-60% of perf. capacity

After getting used to this for two to three weeks, you do more than just one set of each individual exercise. You do this by adding one set of the individual following exercise during each training unit until you do two sets of each exercise.

This is the according supplement for the training sessions after the acclimatisation phase:

Exercises	Time/Sets	Intensity/Reps.	Recommendations
II Steadiness			
Pelvic swing	2 Sets	10 times	no resistance
Pelvic lift	1 Set	10 times	no resistance
Leg scissors from a			
Prone position	1 Set	12 times	no resistance
Leg press	1 Set	18 times	50% of perf. capacity
Adductor machine	1 Set	13 times	60% of perf. capacity
Reverse crunches	1 Set	15 times	no resistance
Crunches	1 Set	20 times	no resistance

The circulation program remains the same for right now.
In the next training session this is what your program would look like:

Exercises	Time/Sets	Intensity/Reps.	Recommendations
II Steadiness			
Pelvic swing	2 Sets	10 times	no resistance
Pelvic lift	2 Sets	10 times	no resistance
Leg scissors from a			
prone position	1 Set	12 times	no resistance
Leg press	1 Set	18 times	50% of max. weight
Adductor machine	1 Set	13 times	60% of max. weight
Reverse crunches	1 Set	15 times	no resistance
Crunches	1 Set	20 times	no resistance

Until you have reached this training volume:

Exercises	Time/Sets	Intensity/Recept..	Recommendations
II Steadiness			
Pelvic swing	2 Sets	10 times	no resistance
Pelvic lift	2 Sets	10 times	no resistance
Leg scissors from a			
prone position	2 Sets	18 times	50% of max. weight
Leg press	2 Sets	18 times	50% of max. weight
Adductor machine	2 Sets	13 times	60% of max. weight
Reverse crunches	2 Sets	15 times	no resistance
Crunches	2 Sets	20 times	no resistance

Keep this program for training your steadiness. Now the changes in the circulation program follow:

Instead of doing the power phase for 30 seconds, increase this time to 40 seconds.

Your first changed training plan would look like this:

Exercises	Time/Sets	Intensity/Reps.	Recommendations
III Circulation			
Recumbent bicycle	2 min	low intensity	50-60% of perf. capacity
Recumbent bicycle	40 sec	high intensity	85-90% of perf. capacity

Recumbent bicycle	3:30 min	low intensity	50% of perf. capacity
Recumbent bicycle	30 sec	high intensity	85-90% of perf. capacity
Recumbent bicycle	3:30 min	low intensity	50% of perf. capacity
Recumbent bicycle	30 sec	high intensity	85-90% of perf. capacity

If you can handle this program well, an increase of the next power phase follows. Then your training program would look like this:

Exercises	Time/Sets	Intensity/Reps.	Recommendations
III Circulation			
Recumbent bicycle	2 min	low intensity	50-60% of perf. capacity
Recumbent bicycle	40 sec	high intensity	85-90% of perf. capacity
Recumbent bicycle	3:30 min	low intensity	50% of perf. capacity
Recumbent bicycle	40 sec	high intensity	85-90% of perf. capacity
Recumbent bicycle	3:30 min	low intensity	50% of perf. capacity
Recumbent bicycle	30 sec	high intensity	85-90% of perf. capacity

and so on until all power phases would be increased to 40 seconds.

If you can handle this program without any problems, increase the training sets for steadiness – as described before – one after another to three.

The circulation training can be extended to 50 seconds later on and if you can handle this completely, you can increase the duration during the power phases one after the other to 60 seconds.

This is how a complete training would look like then:

Exercises	Time/Sets	Intensity/Reps.	Recommendations
I Warm-up			
Recumbent bicycle	10 min.	low intensity	50-60% of perf. capacity
II Steadiness			
Pelvic swing	3 Sets	10 times	no resistance
Pelvic lift	3 Sets	10 times	no resistance

Leg scissors from a prone position	3 Sets	12 times	no resistance
Leg press	3 Sets	18 times	50% of the max. weight
Adductor machine	3 Sets	13 times	60% of the max. weight
Reverse crunches	3 Sets	15 times	no resistance
Crunches	3 Sets	20 times	no resistance

Exercises	Time/Sets	Intensity/Reps.	Recommendations
III Circulation			
Recumbent bicycle	2 min	low intensity	50-60% of perf. capacity
Recumbent bicycle	60 sec	high intensity	85-90% of perf. capacity
Recumbent bicycle	3:30 min	low intensity	50% of perf. capacity
Recumbent bicycle	60 sec	high intensity	85-90% of perf. capacity
Recumbent bicycle	3:30 min	low intensity	50% of perf. capacity
Recumbent bicycle	60 sec	high intensity	85-90% of perf. capacity
IV Cool down			
Recumbent bicycle	6 min	low intensity	50-60% of perf. capacity

Congratulations! You have managed to accomplish a well thought out complete **VigorRobic®** program!

Do this program only for about four to eight weeks. Then you can add bands, foot-weights and other resistances for training your steadiness. Or you may simply include more difficult exercise variations.
You can also add another endurance session to the circulation program so you will get to four power phases.

An important remark to training with weights: If you can easily do 15 (at the bench press 18 or 20 of the exercises for the stomach muscles) repetitions, you have to increase the weight so you will be barely able to do eight repetitions. For the bench press as well as the squat you can probably increase the weight by 5 kg. For other exercises you should increase the weight by an additional 1.25 or 2.5 kg.

9 Training for the Advanced

Are you sure that you grade yourself right? Conditions for this in any case would be that you have consequently completed the training for beginners. You should also be very familiar with the training methods as described before, before you start the program for the advanced.

So: You do have the basic knowledge necessary and an elevated training level: You can "get in"!

Basically it is still valid that we distinguish between training to develop steadiness and training to improve blood circulation. Now the central question is: How do I, who am in an advanced training stage, appropriately increase the intensity of training? The obvious – and correct – answer: by doing the more difficult variations of the known exercises. Furthermore, I recommend for training for steadiness the so-called "training beyond exhaustion".

9.1 Training Beyond Exhaustion

What does training up to exhaustion mean? All sets except for those you do for warm-up should be repeated until the muscles that are being trained with them are so tired that you do not have enough strength to do another complete repetition. This is how far you got in the beginner's program already. Training until failure does get your muscles tired meaning that a further execution of the exercise is not possible anymore but the muscles are not completely exhausted, yet. Mentioned below, you will learn about methods that will make your muscles work beyond the point of exhaustion.

9.1.1 Intensive Repetitions

After you have trained your muscles up to a point of exhaustion, you lower the resistance. If you use disc dumbbells, quickly remove a couple of kilos and then continue the set without a break. As a rule, you can do 2-3 more repetitions. That is quite strenuous! Do you feel the muscles that are being trained? If you do not reduce the weight, you have the possibility of being helped by a training partner. If you do not have the strength to do a repetition yourself, your training partner helps so you will just be able to move the weight upward again. With this help you should be able to do 2-3 more repetitions. The training partner has to adjust his help so much that the intensive repetitions take up all your strength.

When you use bands for your exercises, you simply put them aside and continue the same movement execution without taking a break until you simply cannot continue anymore.

If you are training a difficult exercise variation, you can simply add a couple of repetitions of an easier variation. For example, you lift your pelvis with one leg being stretched out straight into the air (pelvic lift with stretched out leg). When you have reached the point of your muscles failing, you simply put the leg that was stretched out in the air on the ground and now continue to do the exercise in this easier version (pelvic lift). The muscles will start burning!

9.1.2 Principle of the Extended Sets

This means intensifying the intensive repetitions.

For the exercise with weights you need one or even two training partners. During the exercise the weight is reduced. The more the muscles become fatigued, the more weights are removed. Here is a short example of this principle on the leg press:

Put the assigned weights onto the leg press. Use the small disc dumbbells of 2.5 kg for this. After a certain amount of repetition, local muscles start failing. The training partner then quickly removes a couple of discs and you continue the training with a reduced weight without taking a break. If the weight is reduced by 5 kg, you will probably be able to do 3-4 repetitions until the muscles fail again. Then the weight is reduced again and once again you can do 3-4 repetitions. If you want to, you can have the weight reduced again by your partner. What a drudgery! Only do one set with such a high intensity – otherwise there will be the danger of overdoing it.

The same principle can be applied when training with bands. Start with a high resistance of the band and once you get to a point when the muscle is too fatigued, reduce the resistance by simply switching to a band with a lower resistance and so on. This method can be used when exercising without weights or bands as well. Using the example of doing crunches, pick a difficult version at first and after each muscle failure, you switch to an easier exercise as we want to explain the principle again. You start with the variation in which both arms are stretched out behind the head. If you are not able to correctly do the repetitions anymore, move your hands behind the head and when doing so put the elbows to the side. You will notice that now you will be able to do further repetitions. If you get to the point of muscle failure again, cross your arms in front of your chest and continue the exercise without a break. How do your stomach muscles like this?

The method introduced last has a positive effect for the promotion of the circulation as well. Such an intensive method however should only be executed in the last set of your exercise.

9.1.3 Burns

Short, fast partial repetitions are suitable to strain the muscle beyond its momentary failure. 6-12 repetitions of part of the exercise at the end of a set lead to complete fatigue and therefore to strong burns in the working muscles.

This is the way you train: You have accomplished 10 complete repetitions using a certain resistance, a further repetition is not possible anymore. Now you do short, fast part-repetitions until your muscles totally fail. Can you feel the immense burning?

9.2 Training Programs

In this chapter I am introducing some training programs so you will get to know the diversity of the **VigorRobic®** training.

You can combine individual parts of the program or swap them. Add other exercises that were described before or swap individual exercises. There are no limits on how to put together your program as long as you obey the training principles for the increase of steadiness and the circulation with an increased oxygen support.

1. Recommendation:

Exercises	Time/Sets	Intensity/ Reps.	Recommendations
I Warm-up			
Running	10 min	low	50-60% of capacity
II Steadiness			
Squatting with pelvic swing	3 Sets	12 times	band
Pelvic lift with stretching of the lower leg	3 Sets	2 times	foot weight
Leg lift from a prone position	3 Sets	15 times	foot weight
Leg lift with the stretched upper leg while lying on the side	3 Sets	15 times	foot weight
Squat	5 Sets	8 times	70-80% of max. weight
Reverse crunches	3 Sets	20 times	band
Crunches	3 Sets	20 times	disc dumbbell behind the head
III Circulation			
Stepper	3 min	low	50-60% of capacity
Stepper	60 sec	high	85-90% of capacity

Stepper	3:30 min	low	50% of capacity
Stepper	60 sec	high	85-90% of capacity
Stepper	3:30 min	low	50% of capacity
Stepper	60 sec	high	85-90% of capacity
Stepper	3:30 min	low	50% of capacity
Stepper	60 sec	high	85-90% of capacity
IV Cool-down			
Stepper	6 min.	low	50-60% of capacity

2. Recommendation:

Exercises	Time/Sets	Intensity/Reps.	Recommendations
I Warm-up			
Rowing	10 min	low	50-60% of capacity
II Steadiness			
Pelvic swing	3 Sets	10 times	band
Pelvic lift with stretched out leg	3 Sets	12 times	foot weight
Leg scissors while lying on the belly	3 Sets	12 times	foot weight
Lifting the leg from a crawling position	3 Sets	15 times	foot weight
Leg press	2 Sets	12 times	approx. 70 % of max. weight
Adductor machine	3 Sets	15 times	60-70% of the max. weight
Roll-in sideways	3 Sets	20 times per side	disc dumbbell behind the head
Jack-knife	3 Sets	15 times	disc dumbbell behind the head, foot weight,
III Circulation			
Recumbent bicycle	3 min	low	50-60% of capacity
Recumbent bicycle	60 sec	high	85-90% of capacity

Recumbent bicycle	3:30 min	low	50% of capacity
Recumbent bicycle	60 sec	high	85-90% of capacity
Squat	1 Set	8 times	75% of max. weight
Rest interval	3:30 min		
Squat	1 Set	7 times	80% of max. weight
Rest interval	3:30 min		
Squat	1 Set	5 times	85% of max. weight
Rest interval	3:30 min		
Squat	1 Set	4 times	85% of max. weight
IV Cool-down			
Running	6 min	low	50-60% of capacity

3. Recommendation:

Exercises	Time/Sets	Intensity/ Reps.	Recommendations
I Warm-up			
Recumbent bicycle	10 min	low	50-60% of capacity
II Steadiness			
Pelvic lift with knees pressed together	3 Sets	12 times	band
Leg scissors from a prone position	3 Sets	12 times	foot weight
Leg lift while lying on the side, the upper leg is stretched out	3 Sets	10 times	foot weight
Inclined plane	3 Sets	12 times	band
Trunk lift from a prone position	3 Sets	14 times	disc dumbbell behind the head, foot weight
Jackknife	3 Sets	15 times	disc dumbbell behind the head, foot weight
Reverse crunches	3 Sets	20 times	band

III Circulation			
Leg curls with	3 Sets	8 times	approx. 75% of max. weight
Rest interval	3:30 min		
Leg stretch with	3 Sets	8 times	approx. 75% of max. weight
Rest interval	3:30 min		
Leg press	1 Set	8 times	approx. 75% of max. weight
Rest interval	3:30 min		
Squat	1 Set	6 times	approx. 80 % of max. weight
Rest interval	3:30 min		
Squat	1 Set	6 times	approx. 80% of max. weight
Rest interval	3:30 min		
Squat	1 Set	4 times	approx. 85% of max. weight
IV Cool down			
Stepper	6 min	low	50-60% of capacity

10 Training Program Without Any Auxiliary Material

Some of you are not members of a fitness studio. Does that mean that you will not be able to train your potency with **VigorRobic®**? The answer is a definite no! The training principle of **VigorRobic®** also offers the possibility for training without any auxiliary material such as a rowing machine, a stationary bike, training machines, weight cuffs or bands.

Since for the training of the circulation you have only been introduced to exercises using weights or machines, now I additionally introduce "pattering". What is "pattering"? It is a fast running on the spot with a maximum use of the knee and the legs. You have to move your legs as fast as possible. Bend your knees a little as this will increase the strain on the upper thighs – and bend the straight back forward a little *(picture 77)*

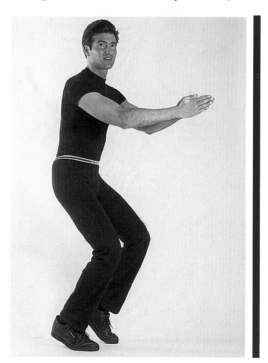

Picture 77

Below I will introduce two training concepts.

First training program

Exercises	Time/Sets	Intensity/Reps.	Recommendations
I Warm-up Running on the spot	5-10 min	low	50-60% of capacity
II Steadiness Squat with pelvic swing	3 Sets	12 times	Flex your muscles when you are in the final positon
Little pelvic lift with leg lift	3 Sets	10 times	
Leg lift from a prone position	3 Sets	12 times	
Leg lift while lying on the side	3 Sets	15 times	Do not forget the tension!
Reverse crunches	3 Sets	20 times	
Crunches	3 Sets	20 times	
III Circulation Running on the spot	3 min	low	50-60% of capacity
Pattering	60 sec	high	85-90% of capacity
Running on the spot	3:30 min	low	50% of capacity
Pattering	60 sec	high	85-90% of capacity
Running on the spot	3:30 min	low	50 % of capacity
Pattering	60 sec	high	85-90% of capacity
Running on the spot	3:30 min	low	50% of capacity
Pattering	60 sec	high	85-90% of capacity
IV Cool-down Running on the spot	5-7 min	low	50-60% of capacity

Second Training Program

Exercises	Time/Sets	Intensity/Reps.	Recommendations
I Warm-up			
Running on the spot	5-10 min	low	50-60% of capacity
II Steadiness			
Little pelvic lift	3 Sets	15 times	
Pelvic lift with foot lift	2 Sets		12 times
Leg scissors from a prone position	3 Sets	15 times	
Leg lift while lying on the side with stretched out Upper leg	3 Sets	15 times	
Leg lift while standing on hands and knees	2 Sets	12 times	
Jack-knife	4 Sets	20 times	
III Circulation			
Pattering	45 sec	high	85-90% of capacity
Running on the spot	3:30 min	low	50% of capacity
Pattering	45 sec	high	85-90% of capacity
Running on the spot	3:30 min	low	50% of capacity
Pattering	45 sec	high	85-90% of capacity
Running on the spot	3:30 min	low	50% of capacity
Pattering	80 sec	high	85-90% of capacity
Running on the spot	3:30 min	low	50% of capacity
Pattering	80 sec	high	85-90% of capacity
IV Cool-down			
Running on the spot	5-7 min	low	50-60% of capacity

You can substitute the exercises mentioned here by others or change the times in the circulation program depending on your readiness for performance. The only thing that is important is – and this I cannot emphasise on often enough – that the basic training rules for steadiness and circulation are considered when putting together your individual **VigorRobic®** program.

11 The 8-12 Minute Program for Training at Home

Finally I want to show a possibility to those who say that they do not have any time for training of how they can concentrate on training their potency in only 8-12 minutes training a day. You do have 8-12 minutes, don't you? At least this much for your virility should be worth it to you. You could, for example, get up 10 minutes earlier or go to bed a little bit later. Your body will thank you for it! And please pay attention to this:

You take turns training for steadiness and for circulation on different days.

Here finally is a complete training program for men who have little time.

1 Day "Steadiness"

Exercises	Time/Sets	Intensity/ Reps.	Recommendations
I Warm-up Running on the spot	2-3 min	low	50-60% of capacity
II Steadiness Pelvic swing	1 Set	15 times	In the final position tighten your muscles and hold this position.
Pelvic lift	2 Sets	15 times	Just like in the exercise before, but press your knees together in addition to that.
Leg scissors from a prone position	1 Set	15 times	Do not forget the tension!
Pelvic lift with stretched out lower leg	1 Set	15 times	Keep the leg stretched out the whole time.

Leg lift while lying on the side with a stretched Upper leg	1 Set	15 times	Change sides after 15 repetitions.
Jack-knife	2 Sets	20 times	The muscle training is completed with this.
III Cool-down Running	2-3 min	low	50-60% of capacity

2. Day "Circulation"

Exercises	Time/Sets	Intensity/ Reps.	Recommendations
I Warm-up Running on the spot	2-3 min	low	50-60% of capacity
II Circulation Pattering	45 sec	high	85-90% of capacity
Running	3:30 min	low	50% of capacity
Pattering	45 sec	high	85-90% of capacity
Running	3:30 min	low	50% of capacity
Pattering	45 sec	high	85-90% of capacity
III Cool down Running	1-2 min	low	50-60% of capacity

This is a short program. But daily training makes it effective. I want to remark as a little hint, that wearing foot cuffs when training for steadiness as well as when pattering increases the intensity.

Perhaps you can add resistances for the training for steadiness, for example a band. The short training will become more intensive at any rate then!

I wish you

- lasting endurance
- good success
- and last but not least lots of fun

with **VigorRobic**®·

Epilogue

Medical-Scientific Foundations/Basics of VigorRobic® Training

VigorRobic® differs from other – more or less fashionable – training programs especially because it was not developed to find a new take-off to improve the physical fitness.

VigorRobic® rather is a logical and practical training conversion of a special branch of scientific research over a couple of years with the goal to be able to treat certain insufficiencies effectively.

The medical-scientific background should be described at least roughly and made available to people who are interested in it by giving references to my related publishings in different special branches of this topic.

Increase of the Oxygen Support and Increase of the Inflow of Blood by VigorRobic® Training

For the first time – all over the world – a new method was developed with the help of which the amount of oxygen and by this the blood circulation in the penis do not have to be measured invasively, meaning some medical instruments have to be inserted into the body. An oxygen sensor electrode was attached to the glans of penis and due to certain electronic-chemical processes it was possible then to measure the oxygen concentration so we were able to get according figures from voluntary candidates.

I have published the results of this scientific examination in the largest European scientific periodical for urology, the "British Journal of Urology (83,1998). Further measurements followed with the question of the change of circulation and amount of oxygen in the penis during sports activities; the results I have published in the scientific periodical "Medicine and Science in Sports and Exercise" (31:5 supplement, 1999).

The effectiveness of the different **VigorRobic®** exercises that are described in chapter 7.1 and 7.2 of this book, I have also verified by exact measurements of the change in blood circulation on voluntary candidates during the exercises. For all of these exercises – executed as described in the mentioned chapters, an increase of circulation in the penis was proven.

A part of the data can be read in the most renowned scientific periodical "The Journal of Urology (162:4, 1999). Further publications in scientific periodicals about the effect that **VigorRobic®** exercises have on the circulation and the oxygen soon will follow in the German as well as in the English language in the near future.

Some of the candidates even had the build-up of pressure in the penis measured while they were doing the **VigorRobic®** exercises. This was done by inserting the measuring instrument right in the cavernous body of the penis under sterile surgical circumstances (caversonometry). This way I was able to prove the increase of muscular activities as well as the contemporary increase of pressure in the penis.

A publication of this scientifically obtained data is planned.

Delaying the Ejaculation With the Help of VigorRobic® Training

Some of the patients who visited my urology consultation hours complained about getting a too "quick" ejaculation. I prescribed the VigorRobic program, especially the exercises from chapter 6.

With the help of objective data I was able to prove that after doing the training program for 12 weeks the problems clearly became fewer, meaning the ejaculation was delayed.

You can read the patients' data before the **VigorRobic®** training in the German-language scientific periodical "Der Urologe" (The Urologist) (38:1, 1999). The data that was gathered after doing the **VigorRobic®** program will be published shortly.

Photo & Illustration Credits

Cover Photo: Bongarts Sportfotografie GmbH, Hamburg
Photos: Anita Wenger, Cologne
Illustrations: Miriam Knupper, Rösrath
Cover Design: Birgit Engelen

Tips for Success

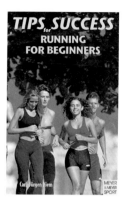

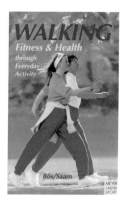

Carl-Jürgen Diem
**Tips for Success –
Running for Beginners**

This book gives the running beginner helpful hints for all questions related to running. It offers information about the form and volume of training as well as clothing and nutrition, and is also a good source of advice for the more experienced runner. It gives practical advice for all those who want to start running as well as for coaches and instructors.

104 pages
Two-colour print
Illustrations
Paperback, 11.5 x 18 cm
ISBN 1-84126-072-X
£ 6.95 UK/$ 9.95 US/
$ 12.95 CDN/€ 9.90

Klaus Bös/Joachim Saam
Walking
Fitness & Health
through Everyday Activity

Walking is introduced as an especially health-promoting kind of sport, which anyone can indulge in. This book describes the basics of walking technique, considers the necessary clothing, the appropriate medical background, and also gives advice on diet. It provides interesting incentives for the professional as well as the beginner, like schemes for strengthening the whole body or tips for new kinds of walking e.g. body walking (meditative walking).

112 pages, 20 photos
Paperback, 11.5 x 18 cm
ISBN 1-84126-001-0
£ 5.95 UK/$ 8.95 US/
$ 12.95 CDN/€ 9.90

MEYER
&MEYER
SPORT

MEYER & MEYER Verlag | Von-Coels-Straße 390 | D-52080 Aachen, Germany | Fax +49 (0)2 41-9 58 10-10

Tips for
Success

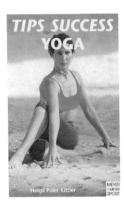

Helga Polet-Kittler
Tips for Success – Yoga

The present book describes a
one-month schedule, including
exercises for each day. It is
highly suited to people who wish
to practice yoga in the home,
in groups or associations, as
well as in sport and fitness
centres. It also provides
valuable tips and directions to
trainers and course instructors.

About 120 pages
4 photos, 135 illustrations
Paperback, 11.5 x 18 cm
ISBN 1-84126-081-9
£ 6.95 UK/$ 9.95 US/
$ 12.95 CDN/€ 9.90

MEYER & MEYER Verlag | Von-Coels-Straße 390 | D-52080 Aachen, Germany | Fax +49 (0)2 41 - 9 58 10 -10